THE GRACIE DIET

THE GRACIE DIET

The Secret of the Champions

Rorion Gracie

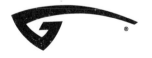

Gracie Publications

Copyright © 2010 by Rorion Gracie.
Second Edition 2017
First published in 2010 by Gracie Publications.
All rights reserved. No part of this publication may be reproduced, stored in a retrieval system, or transmitted in any form or by any means, electronic, mechanical, photocopying, recording, scanning, or otherwise, without the prior written permission of the copyright owner.

DISCLAIMER
Limitation of Liability/Disclaimer of Warranty: While the publisher and author have used their best efforts in preparing this book, they make no representations or warranties with respect to the accuracy or completeness of the contents of this book and specifically disclaim any express or implied warranties. Please note that the information and advice given on and in this book are not intended as a substitute for medical advice. Always consult your doctor or physician before you begin any diet or weight loss program. The author and publisher, and any affiliated websites, subsidiary, person or representative of either party, including Rorion Gracie, shall in no event be held liable to any party for any direct, indirect, punitive, special, incidental or other consequential damages arising directly or indirectly from any use of this material, which is provided "as is," and without warranties.

Library of Congress
Gracie, Rorion – The Gracie Diet

PCN Number: 2010915389

ISBN: 978-0-9759411-0-2

Gracie Publications
3515 Artesia Boulevard
Torrance, CA 90504 - USA
www.GraciePublications.com

Printed in the USA

To Uncle Carlos

CONTENTS

Foreword by Romeu Fadul Junior, M.D. 9
Introduction 12

PART ONE – THE GRACIE DIET

Chapter 1:
Origins of the Gracie Diet 20
Your Food Determines the Quality of Your Life 22
Dietary Decisions 24

Chapter 2:
The Food Industry Isn't Interested in Your Health 29
Stories of the Gracie Diet's Healing Powers 31
You Have Nothing to Lose and Everything to Gain 33
The Secret is Proper Food Combinations and Spacing Meals 36

Chapter 3:
Where Are You Now? 40
Establish a Base Point 40

Chapter 4:
The Hard Part: Changing Your Eating Habits 51
The Belt Graduation System 52
Your Current Eating Habits 55
Your First Meal the Gracie Way 58

Chapter 5:
Getting Started 62
Make Healthy Eating Into a Habit 63
Changing Habits Requires a Plan 64
Reviewing the Basic Concepts 65

PART TWO – USING THE GRACIE DIET

Chapter 6:
A Family Affair 70
The Power of Example 70
A Quick and Simple Way to Kick the Junk Food Habit 72
What to Do When Kids Demand Junk Food 73
The Ultimate Halloween Trick 73
Birthdays and Other Parties 74
How to Win the Kids Over, One Bite at a Time 74

Chapter 7:
Don't Be Afraid to Ask for the Best 77
Your Guide to Food Combinations 79
The Gracie Diet Table 80

Chapter 8:
How to Eat Healthily When You're on the Run 86
Learn the Food Selection Process 87
How Well Do You Know the Combinations? 89
Real Life Examples Drawn from
the Menus of Popular Restaurants 94

Chapter 9:
Detox the Gracie Way 103
Fasting 103
The Lime Regimen 105
The Cleansing Program 106
Obstipation 108
The Digestive Process 108

Chapter 10:
Tips for Losing Weight 113
How to Acquire the Gracie "Iron Will" 113
Calorie Control 114
Play This Game at Your Next Meal 114
A Surefire Way to Burn Fat 115
Managing Your Carbohydrates 115
Protein Sources 116
Fat Facts 117
How to Lose Weight and Still Occasionally Enjoy Alcohol 117

Chapter 11:
The Role of Exercise 120
Make It Fun 121
Start Slowly 122
Keep Climbing 122

Chapter 12:
Final Considerations 126
The Gracie Diet 14-Day Meal Plan 129
Entrées Menu Index 138

FOREWORD

Health – it is first and foremost in our lives, and so it is the first word in this book. In medicine, as in the martial art of jiu-jitsu, the masters pass to us the "secrets" they've learned through years of practice and experience. Then, we pass this knowledge to the next generation to propagate the science, and the sport, for the benefit of all. This passage of knowledge is especially effective when handed down from parent to child. In the context of family life, the child explores, reinforces, and refines these experiences on a daily basis leading to a deeper understanding and appreciation of the lessons. I commend Grand Master Rorion Gracie, one of the leading representatives of the most complete form of self-defense, for seeking to transform the world into a healthier place by sharing the dietary lessons he learned from over 85 years of his family's research.

We fill our busy lives with work and play, but pay little attention to daily nutrition and the consequences of our eating habits – even though it's the most important aspect of our lives. Medical evidence has shown that acidic diets are bad for your health as well as the possible cause for a variety of diseases. Grand Master Carlos Gracie, Rorion's uncle, confirmed this through his own experience. In response, he developed a diet to counter the ill-effects of acidic eating habits. The empirical evidence of several decades of positive results proves the Gracie Diet helps to keep the body healthy, young, and full of energy, and contributes to the reversal of illnesses such as irritable bowel syndrome, gastritis, and diabetes. Today, his entire family and their thousands of students and followers follow the diet and are helping to spread to the word.

Rorion changed the way the world looked at martial arts by creating the UFC to showcase the supremacy of Gracie Jiu-Jitsu as a self-defense system. Today, armed forces, police departments, and countless law enforcement agencies have integrated the techniques into their defensive tactics programs and hundreds of thousands of people practice the family's martial art in schools throughout the world. Rorion now brings the same drive and motivation that revolutionized martial arts to the task of improving the world's eating habits. This book is the foundation of his effort.

"Genius" was the word that came to mind when I first read *The Gracie Diet*, for it gathered in one book 85 years of knowledge, history, clinical tests, and positive results, geared towards improving one's physical and mental health. The Gracie Diet relies on the power of proper food combinations to prevent and even reverse illness as evidenced by the experiences of thousands of followers regardless of nationality, gender, race, religion, or income level.

It has been almost four years since I met Rorion and he introduced me to the Diet over some good açaí. My first impression was that the Diet was too complex and that I lacked the time to read the book and watch his internet videos. But, I was wrong. The Diet is extremely simple with solid and well-defined concepts; and it only took one step to get started!

Rorion borrowed the belt system from jiu-jitsu to motivate progress. Starting as a white belt, I gradually increased my knowledge and understanding. Within a few weeks, I was a black belt and eager to share the positive results of my experience! This book was the ally I needed to move from dietary inertia to embrace life-changing daily eating habits. You can do it, too.

Your transformation will require study and repetition of the teachings, and that requires an open mind and dedication. To read about a theory is one thing, but to connect yourself to it through practice is a different story. Simply reading this book will not change your life, but it is the first step. This book will stimulate you to practice the daily teachings and ultimately improve your health and enable you to achieve your goals.

Romeu Fadul Junior, M.D.

INTRODUCTION

I came to America in the 1970s with a dream – to establish my family's Brazilian style of jiu-jitsu as the most effective self-defense system in the world. To prove my point, I challenged anyone – regardless of size, weight, athleticism, or martial arts skill – to defeat me in one-on-one, no-holds-barred combat. I quickly convinced the martial arts community in Southern California that the Gracie system was amazingly effective. In 1993, I co-created the Ultimate Fighting Championship® to showcase my family's art against all-comers. In the beginning, the UFC was a pay-per-view extravaganza that pitted all varieties of martial arts against each other in the first modern fighting competition without rules, judges, or time limits. The repeated victories of the Gracie Jiu-Jitsu practitioner against larger, stronger, and highly skilled fighters sparked a revolution in the martial arts world that has continued to this day. Today, the UFC is the leading venue for the fastest growing sport on the planet. Despite the implementation of rules, time limits, and weight classes, Brazilian jiu-jitsu continues to be the essential skill for surviving in the octagon and in the street. It is the martial art of choice for U.S. Army and countless other military and law enforcement agencies. I have fulfilled that dream.

Now, I have an even greater task. My new mission is to expand the concept of self-defense beyond physical combat to include lifestyle changes that will enable you to defeat the enemy within. That's self-defense in the fullest meaning of the term. Millions of Americans struggle with the health challenges related to diet and weight control. The United States spends more money on healthcare than any other country, yet it is the most obese nation in history, where childhood obesity is epidemic, and poor nutrition is increasing the rates of heart disease, diabetes, and cancer. In the face of these alarming trends, many people simply surrender just as they would if facing an attacker twice their size. In much the same way that Gracie Jiu-Jitsu revolutionized thinking about physical combat, I believe the Gracie Diet will revolutionize your thinking about healthy eating habits and help you win the fight against internal assailants such as obesity, lack of energy, and a variety of health problems. I promise you can do it! Reading this book is the first step toward leading a healthier, more energetic life. In the pages that follow you'll find very specific, highly practical guidelines for optimizing your eating habits, controlling your weight, and maintaining that control for the rest of your life. In fact, as time passes, you'll find the routine becomes easier. As in jiu-jitsu, it's just a matter of consistently using the tools and techniques you've learned. But before you can start using those techniques, there are a few key principles you must understand.

First and foremost, you must embrace the basic metaphor of this book: Weight control is a matter of defending yourself in a fight against a ruthless opponent who will use every trick in the book to harm you. Of course, we both know that there really is no external enemy. The person who is eating unhealthy foods is the same person who's suffering the consequences. That's you. But for reasons that will become clear as we move ahead, it's important to start separating your negative, self-destructive impulses from the authentic "you" who wants a healthy and fulfilling life. This is really important, so let's look closely at exactly what it means. Imagine that you're waiting in the checkout line of a supermarket – a perfect location to get mugged by unhealthy eating, just like a dark alley at midnight is a good place to get mugged by a thief. You've been walking the aisles looking at food for an hour or more. You're hungry – and maybe a little tired after a long day at work. So many choices and it's all so tasty! If you're like most people, some of your choices (maybe most of them) won't be the healthiest ones. So what? Why not? Don't you deserve a little enjoyment in life? So, you load up the soft drinks, snacks, comfort foods, and you're ready to go home.

But, you're not done yet – there's the checkout line. You're tired. You're tense. And, you're even hungrier now that you've been looking at food for hours. There's the annoying guy with a full shopping cart in front of you. There's the chattering cash register that's going to hit you up for plenty of money. There's the rack full of tabloids with one depressing story after another. You feel guilty for being interested in them, just like you feel guilty for some of the foods you've chosen. Why didn't you get in the other line? It's always so much faster. But wait. It's not all bad. There's a rack full of candy bars – just what you need to soothe your hunger and stress and to give you a quick energy boost…a life raft that will get you through this shipwreck of a checkout line. One of the candies really is a "Lifesaver!" So you grab a pack of Lifesavers® along with a Snickers® or an Almond Joy®. Life is good.

I think you get the picture. So now let's rewind the tape and play back the supermarket scenario from a self-defense perspective. When you entered the supermarket, you entered the arena of mortal combat – and your enemy within was there waiting for you. That opponent has a thousand and one kicks, punches, and dirty tricks that he's ready and willing to use. Your opponent has a punch called, "What's the use?" He has a high kick called, "It's too late to change." He has an arm bar called, "Only a box of Oreo® cookies will stop the pain." These are powerful moves – and your opponent won't be satisfied if you simply surrender. Your opponent wants to kill you. The good news is that I have a counter for all of your opponent's attacks. In this book, I will show you how to defeat that opponent no matter how big and strong he is, or how many fights you've lost to him in the past.

Let's start by clarifying expectations about what you can achieve with this diet continuing with the self-defense metaphor. Some martial arts claim that they can enable anybody to overcome any adversary, no matter how dangerous or formidable, in very little time and without much training.

This was the fantasy behind the ads that appeared in comic books fifty years ago. Who knows how many kids mailed away their allowances to learn the secret moves that could defeat all bullies. All they really got was a false sense of security and a serious misunderstanding of what effective self-defense training really involved. On the other end of the spectrum are those who refuse to believe that any amount of knowledge or training will enable them to survive an attack against a much larger, stronger adversary. At best, these skeptics acknowledge that the techniques might work in training, but don't believe they would work in a real fight.

Do either one of these viewpoints express your feelings about diet and weight control? Do you expect that this book will provide a quick fix – a silver bullet that will resolve your problems in the hour or so that's needed to read it from cover to cover? Or, do you simply dismiss it as yet another one of the hundreds, if not thousands, of fad diet books that will have come and gone over the years? Have you reached the point at which any diet advice is just too little, too late, or too difficult to bring about real change? Both of these extremes echo the voice of your enemy within – and listening to either one of them will prevent you from achieving your dietary objectives.

Here are your first counterattacks. First, give yourself time. It's unlikely that you became overweight or underweight overnight. These conditions usually develop over months or years of poor eating habits. It will take time to reverse the conditions. The Gracie Diet will resolve the problems – but it will take more than a day or a week. Just as you can't instantly defend yourself against a strong-arm robber who is twice your size, you won't defeat this opponent in the time it takes to read the book. Success, in both situations, requires patience and discipline. The Gracie Diet is not a quick weight-loss program. It is not a fad diet or even a restrictive one. In fact, it should not even be called a "diet" since it does not prohibit eating anything.

The Gracie Diet is about education and reprogramming your eating habits. As you restructure your eating habits, a healthy diet will naturally become part of your way of life, as it has been for four generations of the Gracie family, and an ever growing number of people around the world.

My uncle, Carlos Gracie, developed this concept based on his observations of the effects of various food combinations. His original purpose was to ensure that all family members were ready to uphold the Gracie name in an unarmed fight with anyone, anywhere, and at any time. Uncle Carlos was not a doctor. He was a self-taught nutritionist who studied the writings of health experts. From these writings, he drew his own conclusions about the principles of healthy eating. Using himself and the rest of the Gracie family as participants in an experiment that lasted more than 65 years, he was able to fine tune and empirically validate his conclusions.

I want to be very clear about the fact that, like my uncle, I am neither a medical doctor nor a credentialed nutritionist. However, my own health, my family's health, and the health of thousands of individuals around the globe, testify to its benefits. For over eight decades, the dinner table has been our science lab, and the longevity and good health of those who have followed the Gracie Diet is all the evidence I need to know that it works. Fad diets come and go. Every year we see some new program promise to solve weight problems, lower cholesterol, improve heart function, and gastro-intestinal issues, and so on. Some of the diets produce short-term results but none of them stand the test of time. As a result, none of these diets can document long-term benefits. I know of no other regimen except the Gracie Diet that can point to more than 80 years of real life testing and great results.

When I was growing up, I was often told that following the Gracie Diet would pay off after I turned 50. I'm now 65 years old. I base my certainty in the principles of our diet on some simple facts. I am free from most of the health problems that plague many people my age. I'm still able to do the same physical activities, and wear the same size pants I wore forty years ago. I can even keep up with my ten children...and the 8 year old only stops when he's sleeping!

In the 1930s when Uncle Carlos was in the early stages of his research, he pioneered the "self-defense" approach to health issues. He looked at people suffering from different complaints as if they were jiu-jitsu students and characterized their health problems as challenging opponents. My mother, for example, suffered from Irritable Bowel Syndrome. When this healthier way of eating healed her, she became a firm believer in the Gracie Diet. Gradually, my Uncle Carlos began building an almost magical reputation for helping people by modifying their eating habits.

I grew up watching Uncle Carlos and my father live long and healthy lives. They knew this was made possible by the Gracie Diet, and before I knew it the Diet became a way of life for me as well. I learned to prioritize the importance of what I ate because I knew each meal had a direct impact on my health. In the pages that follow, I'll teach you the strategies and tactics that I've embraced. I'll be "in your corner" at every meal. Just as I've taught chokes and arm locks to defeat any adversary, I'll train you in "dietary self-defense."

You'll learn to avoid certain combinations of foods – even some that give you pleasure – because you know they're not good for you. You'll learn the effect that self-discipline – or the lack thereof – will have on your life and on the lives of your loved ones. Although the reputation of our family is a result of our sensational accomplishments in the ring, our healthy eating habits made this possible by maximizing the potential of the Gracie warriors. Truly, the Gracie Diet has been our secret weapon. Now, it's your turn to learn the secrets.

R.G.

PART ONE:

The Gracie Diet

CHAPTER 1:

"The beginning is the most important part of the work."
                                    - Plato

Origins of the Gracie Diet
Around 1914, a Japanese jiu-jitsu champion named Mitsuyo Maeda immigrated to Brazil. There, he met my grandfather, Gastão Gracie, a Brazilian scholar and businessman. Gastão helped Maeda settle in the new country, and in return Maeda taught jiu-jitsu to Carlos, my grandfather's oldest son. When the family moved to Rio de Janeiro in the early 1920s, Carlos, still in his teens, decided to teach jiu-jitsu. In order to promote his school, he issued open challenges to anyone who wanted a match. Over time, Carlos introduced his brothers to jiu-jitsu and they too became totally dedicated to the art. So, around 1925, they opened the first Gracie Jiu-Jitsu Academy.

My father, Helio Gracie, was the youngest of the brothers. Due to his frail health, his doctors recommended that he limit his physical activity. Helio spent the next few years watching his brothers practicing. One day, one of his brothers was late for a class, so Helio, who was only sixteen at the time, offered to teach the lesson. The student was so impressed that he chose Helio to be his new teacher. Helio began experimenting with different ways to apply the traditional Japanese techniques. By focusing on leverage, timing, and natural body movements, he found that he could increase the effectiveness of many of the techniques and make them work against much bigger and stronger opponents. Helio dissected and tested every move until he discovered how to make it work against virtually any opponent

– he literally reinvented the Japanese martial art. Soon, he too was challenging all kinds of opponents to fight anytime and anywhere. Helio's unexpected victories catapulted him to stardom; he became the first sports legend in Brazilian history and came to be known as the father of Brazilian jiu-jitsu.

It was only when his brothers started demonstrating their abilities on the mat that Carlos, then in his late 20s, shifted his focus and found his true calling in life. He immersed himself in a variety of subjects related to body, mind, and spirit. His studies in philosophy, religion, and health established him as the spiritual leader of the Gracie family.

Since none of the Gracie brothers were physically gifted, they had to stay healthy in order to sustain the open challenge that had become the family hallmark. My father told me that in the old days, tough guys would knock on their door at ten o'clock at night, to test themselves against one of the Gracies. He had to get out of bed, defeat the challenger, and then go back to sleep! Optimal health was essential. This is what motivated Carlos to study the links between diet and physical performance. He began his research by reading a wide range of opinions from various health experts and nutritionists. Then, he narrowed his interest to food combining, which he saw as the most important aspect of nutrition. Eventually, he also studied the use of medicinal herbs.

I based this book on the diet principles that my Uncle Carlos discovered and that my family has followed for many years. I supplemented those principles with my own experience as an athlete, a parent, and a teacher. I'm certainly aware of the great number and variety of diet books on the market covering nearly every approach to eating. In fact, if someone were to publish a book suggesting that we shouldn't change anything in our eating habits, it might be a bestseller! But, I'm confident this book is like no other.

Your Food Determines the Quality of Your Life

Simply put, your food determines the quality of your life. It determines not just how you feel from day to day, but also how long you will live, how well you will live, and possibly how you will eventually die. It's common knowledge that unhealthy eating habits contribute to chronic illnesses or, at the very least, can result in obesity, malnutrition, or other imbalances that threaten your health. So remember, everything you eat or drink, will either improve or diminish your health. A poor diet can also seriously affect your mental and emotional health.

Michael D. Gershon, M.D., Professor and Chairman, Department of Anatomy and Cell Biology, New York Presbyterian Hospital / Columbia University Medical Center, in his book *The Second Brain* (HarperCollins) explains that the Enteric Nervous System, is like an independent nervous system, specifically designed for executing the intestinal functions, located in the wall of the GI track with 100 million neurons, that produce the neurotransmitters responsible for the communication between the nerve cells. Today, we know that 80% of our immunologic potential is located in the intestinal flora, which reinforces the argument that our defenses and vitality are related to the proper functioning of the intestine. Another interesting discovery is that about 90% of the serotonin (neurotransmitter responsible for the feeling of well-being), is produced in the gut, demonstrating the correlation between these organs with depression. Some experts now believe that Crohn's

Disease, Ulcerative Colitis, Diverticulitis, Diabetes, Constipation, Irritable Bowel Syndrome, and Parkinson's are some of the diseases that could be associated to neurochemical alterations in the intestine, or "the second brain."[1]

The late biochemist and Orthomolecular Medicine specialist from Brazil, Professor Hélion Póvoa, member of the Academia Nacional de Medicina, reinforces this thesis in his book O Cerebro Desconhecido (Objetiva). He wrote, "if the intestines are fine, the brain will be healthy, and it is crucial, that the medical community becomes aware of this, to better orient their patients. If the intestine is not working properly, the tendency is to increase the depression and anxiety, because of the significant amount of serotonin and melatonin produced in that organ."[2]

The inability to participate in recreational activities can lead to isolation from friends and family, and even to depression, and, of course, only accelerates the harmful effects of poor eating habits. I recall hearing an obese father lament, "My son wanted to throw the football but I couldn't get up off the couch." This situation is not only tough for the parent, but also affects the child.

Your eating habits begin to form at birth based on how and what your parents fed you. Essentially, your parents taught you how to eat. And your parents learned how to eat from their parents. I was fortunate to grow up in a family in which healthy eating was taken very seriously. My parents filled my baby bottles with papaya or figs blended with honey, or freshly squeezed watermelon juice blended with bananas and other natural foods. Today, my children's bottles contain the same fresh and nutritious foods – because that's

---

[1] https://www.scientificamerican.com/article/gut-second-brain/
[2] http://medholos.blogspot.com/search?q=H%C3%A9lion+P%C3%B3voa)

what my parents taught me. I'm confident that my children will pass these good habits on to their children.

I realize that not everyone had the benefit of my role models and may have never developed good eating habits. I also know it's difficult to change habits ingrained in your life's routines since birth. But, your life depends on accepting the challenge to change and telling yourself, "That was then, this is now!" This commitment to change your diet and improve the quality of your life is perhaps the most wonderful gift you can give to yourself and your loved ones. That is why it's important to develop good habits as they are as hard to break as the bad ones.

Dietary Decisions

We can learn much about natural eating habits by observing animals in the wild. Animals exhibit very specific eating habits that have evolved over thousands of years. They follow regular and simple diets that keep them healthy. Are there overweight giraffes or zebras? I don't think so. Nor do zebras need Tums®, Kaopectate®, or Metamucil® as long as they stick to their customary foods. Humans, on the other hand, face a more complicated situation. We not only have many more options than zebras or giraffes, but we were blessed with a uniquely powerful decision-making capability and, therefore, must contend with the internal opponent tempting us with unhealthy choices at every turn.

In a fight, an inexperienced person panics in the midst of what they perceive as total chaos. They act out of desperation and play right into the hands of a better-trained adversary. The unschooled fighter simply lacks the tools to win the fight. Their actions not only guarantee their defeat, but can even hasten that outcome. In a fight with a mugger, that can mean leaving yourself open to a punch or a choke. In a fight against the inner opponent, it means making food choices that will undermine your health and well-being. Imagine that your opponent sprinkled an invisible, tasteless poison on a container of ice cream. You would eat it without giving a thought to the deadly consequences. On the other hand, you wouldn't touch the ice cream if you knew of the poison. Just as in the fight against the mugger, your ability to recognize threats and respond with the proper counter will ensure your victory in the battle for your health when making dietary choices.

One of the least known dietary dangers is the negative impact that improper food combining has on your digestive system and overall health. Your inner opponent's most common and most successful tactic is to attack you through your taste buds. Most people simply follow their taste buds and mix foods without giving any thought to the implications of various food combinations. Put simply, taste drives our food selections and even determines the order in which we eat them. For example, many people want a sweet dessert or a fruit after eating a typical American main course comprised of meat, vegetables, and starches. It just seems natural because that's how you ate as a child. The problem is that taste alone can drive us to choose foods that do not digest well together. The result is inefficient digestion, fermentation, and acidity. The effects are real but often subtle, and soon they become part of everyday life. Poor food choices repeated every day, year after year, create an array of health issues which will vary from person to person. Many accept headaches, heartburn, gas, or indigestion as a natural consequence of eating. They take an aspirin or an antacid to eliminate the symptom and think the problem is gone.

Not quite! If you were driving down the highway and a red light began to blink on the panel of your car, would you cover it with a Band-Aid® and keep driving, or would you look for a mechanic to fix the problem? If your answer was to find a mechanic, remember that aspirin and antacid are just like a Band-Aid®! If you would not ignore an alert signal for your vehicle, why would you ignore an alert signal from your body?

Learn to listen to your body. It will tell you when it isn't operating at peak efficiency. The immediate effect of an incompatible food combination may be just a subtle discomfort that varies from person to person. One person may feel a headache, another may have a stomachache, and a third may feel nothing at all. In this book, I'll show you how to recognize the signs of unhealthy food options. To me those signs are very clear, just as the mistakes of an untrained student are obvious when I'm teaching jiu-jitsu. Soon the mistakes will be obvious to you, too. And, so will the right choices. In time, you will find that the Gracie Diet, like Gracie Jiu-Jitsu, will produce maximum results from minimal effort. Specifically, this regimen enables the body to maximize the nutritional benefits of food while using minimal energy to digest it. Your body will function more efficiently and you will feel better and have more energy all of the time.

Is there medical or scientific proof that these combinations are healthy?

Not yet. However, researchers have taken interest in the diet due to positive results in the treatment of a variety of illnesses. Although Carlos Gracie was not a doctor, he diligently studied the works of countless nutritionists, health professionals, and naturalists. These were the sources from which he drew his conclusions. Then, he used himself and the large number of family members as subjects for his research, which lasted more than 65 years. The final objective of any good diet should not be to lose weight or to increase longevity, but, more importantly, to ensure a good quality of life. Observing the long and healthy lives lived by brothers Carlos and Helio Gracie was enough to inspire me to follow in the same path. However, it is the life-changing impact that these eating habits have had on thousands of people, many of whom I have personally coached, that came to be the irrefutable evidence of the benefits of the Gracie Diet.

Points to Remember:
- Everything you eat or drink will either improve or harm your health. Choose wisely!
- Your body uses an incredible amount of energy to digest each meal. Do whatever you can to increase the efficiency of the digestive process.
- Learning to manage the temptations elicited by your taste buds is the first step towards optimizing your health.

> **The Gracie Diet In A Nutshell**
>
> - Wash your hands before every meal.
> - Thoroughly wash all fruits and vegetables before consumption.
> - Peel fruits before you eat them unless you are certain that the skin is free from pesticides.

CHAPTER 2:

"The first wealth is health."

- Ralph Waldo Emerson

The food industry isn't interested in your health, and the pharmaceutical industry thrives on your sickness!
I once met a young woman who won a prize from a national magazine for her original cake recipe. When she entered the contest, she learned that appearance rather than taste would determine the winner. The winning recipe had to look great on the pages of the magazine. After all, readers weren't going to eat the food; they were just going to look at it. So, she baked an amazingly colorful and beautifully shaped lemon cake. It happened to taste bland and was full of unhealthy ingredients, but those same ingredients enhanced the cake's structure and appearance. Her prize was a bicycle.

In a television commercial, breakfast cereal rains down into a bowl in slow motion. In the next shot, milk pours from the sky, followed by beautiful red strawberries that magically land perfectly spaced on the bed of cereal. Then, the cereal box descends to the left of the bowl accompanied by a full glass of orange juice. Wow! It's a perfect breakfast! The message is that any cereal that's so visually attractive probably tastes wonderful too. After all, anything that looks so good and tastes so good must be good for you as well. The emphasis is on visual appeal with the implication that it will also taste good.

Some products tout the health benefits of vitamins. The vitamins found in processed foods are invariably produced in a laboratory. These vitamins differ from those found in natural sources such as fruits, vegetables, or animals. What's the difference? If you drink a large amount of carrot juice, your body will take from it the naturally occurring Vitamin A (beta-carotene) it needs and expel the excess. However, if you take an excess of Vitamin A in highly concentrated forms, you risk overloading your liver, and could suffer from hypervitaminosis.

It is not a coincidence that obesity is at an all-time high in the United States, the country with the most advertising dollars spent by the food industry. You might feel differently if you read the *Los Angeles Times* article (Maugh II, 2008) in which researchers found that "the arteries of many obese children and teenagers are as thick and stiff as those of 45-year-olds." It makes you wonder about the condition of their 45-year-old parents' arteries. That was not the topic of the article, but the implications are clear – just because a food looks good, doesn't mean that it's good for you. To make matters worse, studies now show that sugar is more addictive than cocaine.[3]

Chefs all over the world strive to combine three elements in their meals: visual appeal, enticing aroma, and delicious taste.

"What about the impact of the food on one's health?" I asked a renowned chef in a high-end restaurant.

He replied, "Well, that's not a priority, although I always use the best ingredients. Eating should be a pleasant experience, and that is what I want to provide for the guests in my restaurant."

My friend's restaurant is indeed very successful. However, he is quite overweight, has health problems, and is on a

---

[3] Lenoir, Magalie et al. "Intense Sweetness Surpasses Cocaine Reward." Ed. Bernhard Baune. PLoS ONE 2.8 (2007): e698. PMC. Web. 8 Jan. 2017.

strict diet that – for his own good – prevents him from eating the very foods he serves to others.

I was invited to Denmark to lecture on the Gracie Diet at a convention of five hundred very influential chefs. In my speech, I acknowledged that a good meal meant appreciating a beautiful presentation, sensing the aroma, and savoring the taste of every bite. But, I offered the most important part of a good meal was feeling light and comfortable after eating! I challenged the chefs, in keeping with the family tradition, by stating:

> As some of the most influential chefs of the international cuisine, I am sure you are constantly visiting different restaurants as part of your research, to find new flavors, and develop new ideas. That said, I am willing to bet that, if any of you go to your favorite restaurant, to order the most expensive plate, followed by the most elaborate dessert in the menu, by the time you get home, you will not be feeling well.

Many nodded in agreement and one later confided, "Rorion, I have no doubt that chefs like us are poisoning the population."

The proper food combinations suggested by the Gracie Diet not only allows for tremendous creativity, and delicious taste, but more importantly, it will crown the meal with the sensation of well-being, without the bloating, headache, or acid indigestion that can ruin your sleep.

Stories of the Gracie Diet's Healing Powers

While Carlos was not a doctor, he was a keen observer and a self-taught nutritionist. He earned a reputation as a healer through his successes "curing" an array of health problems using food combination principles. His specialty was gastrointestinal illnesses, and he often said, "No ulcer can resist me for thirty days!" Notably, he even treated the head physician at a renowned ulcer clinic in Rio de Janeiro. The doctor's ulcer was so bad that he scheduled himself for a surgical repair. Carlos convinced him to try the Gracie Diet during the weeks prior to the surgery. He taught the doctor's cook how to prepare healthy food combinations and directed the doctor to not eat for five hours between meals.

The doctor was skeptical. "What about my pain?" he asked. "Everyone knows an ulcer patient needs to drink milk and eat frequently." But Uncle Carlos was firm: "Doctor, with all due respect, I am in charge now." The doctor reluctantly agreed to follow the instructions and promised to report back in a few days. On the fourth day, he very excitedly reported that he had slept through the night for the first time in ages. By the tenth day, the pain was completely gone.

By the end of the second week, the X-ray did not detect any traces of an ulcer. The doctor completed the 28-day program and became a believer in the Gracie Diet.

However, he told Carlos, "I cannot tell you how impressed I am. It's as if some kind of magic was performed before my very own eyes. I will be forever grateful to you. If there is ever anything you need, you can rest assured I will be there for you. The only thing I can never do is publicly admit that I was cured by someone who is not a doctor."

Carlos philosophically replied: "Doctor, I didn't treat you expecting publicity. I wanted to refine my treatment. It was in my best interest as well as yours."

On another occasion, a woman lost all of her teeth in a car crash. A renowned oral surgeon implanted new teeth, but the woman's body rejected the implants. The surgeon asked Carlos to suggest a dietary program that would address the body's reaction to the surgery. Again, Carlos developed an eating regimen that worked when conventional medical procedures were at a loss.

While at a summer home in mountains of Teresópolis outside of Rio de Janeiro, a family friend brought Uncle Carlos some tragic news. He had just learned that his wife had intestinal cancer and wanted advice on how to proceed. The "Mountain Guru," as we affectionately called Carlos, devised a plan.

He said, "Do not tell your wife she has cancer. Tell her that she's fine, but the doctor recommended you urgently implement a radical change in your diet, and that you would very much appreciate if she would accompany you on the program."

Uncle Carlos then prepared a specific regimen for the man's wife. The woman, in her mid-forties at that time, lived until her mid-eighties!

At 39 years old, and tipping the scale at 400 pounds, Jessica was diabetic and plagued with high blood pressure. She spent most days sitting and feeling depressed. Twice weekly she would take her sons to jiu-jitsu lessons, where their instructor, who follows the Diet, would often tell the kids to drink water instead of sodas, and choose fruits and vegetables instead of candy and junk food. Inspired by the youngsters' discipline, patience, determination, and the willingness to improve, Jessica decided to change her life. She began drinking only water. Then, she embraced the Gracie Diet and begin walking regularly. In one year, she lost 182 pounds, is no longer diabetic, and has normal blood pressure. Jessica proclaimed with her now ever-present smile, "I feel alive again, and know the best is yet to come!"

You Have Nothing to Lose and Everything to Gain

Carlos believed that proper food combinations were the key to good health. He based this conclusion on hundreds of observations, although the aforementioned are some of the most dramatic. He also observed that improper food combinations were potentially harmful. You need not accept the full body of Carlos' work, but if you approach the Gracie Diet with an open mind, you'll find that, in just a few weeks, the results will speak for themselves and you'll need no more convincing. One of the first things you'll notice will be an increase in your energy level. You'll also find a decrease in the frequency of headaches, irregular bowel movements, heartburn, and stomachaches that could underlie a chronic health problem with serious consequences.

I can't prove that the Gracie Diet is the best way to eat. I've been challenged on various aspects of the Diet over the years. The critics usually cite a lack of scientific evidence to support our claims or studies on nutrition and health that refute either the general concept of food combining, or more often, our observations on specific food combinations. Some have stated that the Gracie family's remarkable health is attributable to good genes more than good eating habits. Notably, no one has condemned the Diet in its entirety, and most acknowledged that, at worst, it will not harm you. I will say nothing to refute the naysayers other than to cite my own experiences and those of my very large family. After four generations, the Gracie Diet has certainly withstood the test of time. For almost a century, this food combination concept has been the cornerstone of our lifestyle, providing abundant energy and outstanding health for a family that has become a symbol of efficiency in physical combat.

Interestingly, nutritionists are starting to champion many of the same ideas that my uncle had been promoting for decades.

One of the diet's most radical concepts is spacing meals at least four and a half hours apart and only consuming water in between meals. In a randomized crossover study

(*Diabetologia*, 2015) conducted in Prague, Czech Republic, doctors concluded that eating two larger meals a day (breakfast and lunch) is more effective than six smaller meals in a reduced-energy regimen for patients with type 2 diabetes.[4] If this regimen is beneficial for those with diabetes, it can only help those who are not diabetic. It's like suggesting to a person who has a cold to rest, eat healthily, and don't smoke. The advice is just as good for those who do not have a cold.

Anahad O'Connor of the *New York Times* cites a 2009 study documented in the *British Journal of Nutrition* in which two groups had identical daily caloric intake over eight weeks. However, one group ate three times a day, while the other ate six times a day. Both groups lost weight and showed no difference in loss of fat or the control of appetite. Other studies show similar results indicating that eating several small meals, or "grazing," was neither better nor worse than consuming three a day as some nutritionists have suggested.

These are only a few cases, but it's comforting to see that many new discoveries in the field of nutrition, are reinforcing Uncle Carlos' dietary regimen.

I recall Uncle Carlos' reaction to an Alka-Seltzer® commercial that proclaimed: "Eat anything you want! If you have indigestion, take an Alka-Seltzer and you'll feel great!" He responded, "How ridiculous! They encourage you to eat wrong so that they can sell you the illusion of a cure. Why not promote healthy eating instead?" Then he added: "Like the fish, people die through their mouths!"

The human body naturally functions in perfect balance. Don't complicate things by feeding it the wrong foods!

---

[4] https://www.ncbi.nlm.nih.gov/pubmed/24838678

Eating right is easy. All you need is common sense and a willingness to learn some basic concepts for combining food. The purpose of this book is to teach you how to choose your foods and improve your eating habits. Do not be surprised if you find out that you can still eat many of the same foods you now enjoy, as long as you consider what you eat them with. Expect immediate improvements in your overall health!

The Secret is Proper Food Combinations and Spacing Meals
While it's always best to eat high-quality organic foods, it's even more important that you properly combine your foods in each meal. It's not a matter of appearance, aroma, or even taste. Instead, the Diet combines foods to help prevent fermentation and blood acidity during digestion. Foods that "combine" are those that mix in a way that is good for your weight control and overall health. Foods that "do not combine," are those mixtures that make digestion more difficult, and as a result, can undermine attempts to regulate your weight control and negatively affect your general well-being. Proper food combination is what differentiates the Gracie Diet from all others.

Uncle Carlos spent several decades identifying which foods combined and which foods should only be eaten by themselves. He also insisted on allowing at least 4 ½ hours between meals to allow the body time to digest completely the stomach's content. He concluded that food combining and meal spacing were the keys to increasing the body's alkalinity – the principal objective of the Gracie Diet.

Dr. Otto Warburg, Medicine Nobel Prize winner in the early 1900s, suggested that cancer cells "live in hypoxic, very low oxygen, and acidic conditions and produce energy from sugars by fermenting them the way yeast does." He theorized that these low-oxygen and highly-acidic conditions caused cancer. Warburg discovered that cancer cells maintain and thrive in a lower pH. Higher pH, which is alkaline, means higher concentration of oxygen molecules, while lower pH, which is acidic, means lower concentrations of oxygen. From this, he concluded, no disease including cancer can survive in an alkaline body. Dr. Warburg recommends finding a space with clean air and practicing deep breathing exercises for improved health. Add to that a diet based on proper combinations of fruits, vegetables, and proteins to promote your body's alkalinity, and you're on your way to great health!

THE ESSENCE OF THE COMBINATIONS

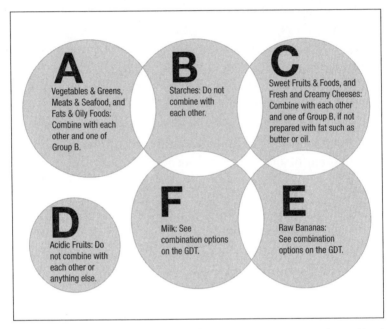

Note: Each intersection in the diagram above represents one properly combined meal possibility. For the complete list of foods and the combination guidelines that govern each group, please reference the Gracie Diet Table on pages 80-82.

Will I have to give up my favorite foods to follow the Diet?
A friend told me that after following the Gracie Diet for a few weeks he was feeling great. Then he decided to go out to dinner and ordered his old favorite dish. The next morning he told me, "My favorite dish made me feel sick all night. I never want to eat it again!" The secret to good health is to learn to like the things that are good for you. Next time you decide you can't resist eating a certain dish, remind yourself that your

> meals shouldn't be determined by taste alone. Make the wise choice! However, if the ingredients of your favorite dish don't combine according to the Gracie Diet, often, the dish can be modified to do so. Besides, who is to say that you can't adopt a new favorite dish?

Points to Remember:
- The essence of the Gracie Diet is proper food combination and spacing meals.
- Drink only water or fresh coconut water between meals.
- Once you start the Gracie Diet, you will notice improvements in your health within two weeks.

 The Gracie Diet In A Nutshell

- Avoid processed juices even if they claim to be 100% natural. A real juice would not last six months on a shelf without preservatives!
- Just because something tastes good, it doesn't mean it's good to eat. Learn to like what is good for you!
- Keep a stock of your favorite fruits and veggies handy. Plan ahead so that you'll have everything you need for your next meal.

CHAPTER 3:

"Your body was created to function perfectly. Don't disturb its natural flow by feeding it incorrectly."

- Helio Gracie

Where Are You Now?
The availability of food determines our diet. Once driven by our ability to hunt, gather, or cultivate, today our food choices are seemingly limitless with nothing to shape our eating habits other than personal preferences and cultural influences. Some people use food as a stress reliever – snacking on chips or drinking a soda much like a bottle calms a baby. Others follow highly restrictive "health food" diets seeking peace of mind in knowing that they are avoiding pesticides, additives, cholesterol, carcinogens, GMOs, and other perceived dangers. In both cases, the experience of eating becomes a form of treatment, like taking medicine. But whether someone is a fast-food addict or a health-food devotee, relatively few people are really aware of what motivates them to eat the way they do.

Establish a Base Point
In order to change, it helps to establish a base point to improve your understanding of your dietary habits. So, let's begin by assessing your current eating and drinking behaviors by evaluating your response to the following thirty questions. A brief discussion of the possible answers follows each question. You may read the discussion prior to answering the questions, but be honest with yourself. Your responses will provide a dietary snapshot of what you eat, when you eat, and how you eat. The results may surprise you as most peo-

ple take this fundamental life behavior for granted based on years of eating habits handed down by parents and shaped by daily routines. If you're not satisfied with your diet and how it makes you feel based on your responses to the questions, then I suggest you give the Gracie Diet a try. You really have nothing to lose as the regimen is easy to follow and you will still be able to eat most of your favorite foods. Reassess your eating habits after you've been following the Diet for a few weeks. You may find your answers have changed as much as your eating habits. Feel free to write your answers in the book, or on a separate sheet of paper.

1. What are your goals for the Gracie Diet?
The way human beings think about what they eat has changed considerably in the last hundred years. Diets consisting of meat, potatoes, and dairy products once defined a healthy meal. We even found virtue in being overweight as it signified the ability to eat well and often. Large physical size also conveyed an image of power and importance. Many of America's wealthiest businessmen were overweight or obese. William Howard Taft, President of the United States from 1909-1913 and later a Justice of the Supreme Court, weighed more than 300 pounds and sometimes needed help getting out of the bathtub. In contrast, we viewed very thin people as poor, weak, and even sickly. Today, we know that excessive fat is unhealthy and it's no longer fashionable. Not surprisingly, the positive views once associated with plumpness are now reserved for thin people. We associate being overweight not only with being unattractive and unhealthy, but also with being poor. In fact, most of America's obese people reside in the nation's poorest regions. Despite the changed attitudes toward excessive weight and the health risks associated with high-fat diets, Americans are still the

world's most obese people.

It's difficult to accept that anyone would work at being unhealthy and physically unattractive. Yet, these are the conditions commonly associated with poor eating habits. On the other hand, you may be satisfied with your current weight and appearance, but how do you feel? Your goals may pertain more to how you feel, rather than how you look. If you're not comfortable with how you look, or how you feel, then do something about it. Making radical changes in your diet won't happen by itself. It will take consistent effort, especially at the beginning. So you'll need worthwhile goals in order to sustain your motivation. Do you have those goals? What are they?

2. What lifestyle changes will your goals require? Are you prepared to make those changes?

The Gracie Diet is more than just a list of foods and how to prepare them. The Diet is really a way of life. Following the Diet means making some real changes – not just in what you eat, but in your whole orientation toward food. And since food is such a basic part of what we do every day, changing your thinking about food really means changing your thinking about your life in general. I can say with total confidence that the changes will be positive ones, but change of any kind doesn't always come easily, especially if you're not well prepared for it.

For example, throughout this book I'll be emphasizing the fact that in order to follow the Gracie Diet, you can no longer decide what to eat simply on the basis of taste. For most people, this is a big change. It means ignoring all those advertisements for fast food hamburgers that have been carefully crafted by expert marketers. It means avoiding the most "taste tempting" items on a restaurant menu, or maybe even avoiding the restaurant itself. Please note, this does not mean you will no longer be able to enjoy delicious meals, you can indeed create delightful food combinations that agree with the Gracie Diet, but you will no longer allow taste to dominate/manipulate your choices in food. You must choose long-term well-being over instant gratification derived from eating unhealthy food. As you begin to change your eating habits, just be aware you're making that choice. As time goes on, you'll know it was the right one.

3. How high is your motivation for reaching your goals?
Success depends on approaching the Diet with a strong sense of motivation that you can sustain over a long period of time. It's normal to start something new with great enthusiasm and excitement. The initial "high" associated with new and different activities frequently fades over time as we hit plateaus in our progress or find the undertaking to be more difficult than expected. Successful progress in both the Diet and in jiu-jitsu relies on having a strong foundation based in part on immediate, sustained positive feedback and on the knowledge that you will win in the long run. Many times a match will seem to be going against us, but the whole orientation of jiu-jitsu training is toward winning in the end, no matter how long it takes. This is why I have been opposed to time limits in sanctioned fights. Jiu-jitsu competitors are motivated for the long haul. There's no time limit for real-life challenges, so there shouldn't be time limits in the most lifelike form of martial arts. Be aware of the difference between excitement and motivation. The main difference is sustainability. Excitement comes and goes – and it always goes eventually. Motivation means "whatever it takes," for an hour, a day, or a lifetime.

4. Who will support you in following the Diet?
Breaking old habits and forming new ones is difficult. The support of family and friends can help with the transition. Changing eating habits is especially difficult because often your routine is tied to factors beyond your direct control – like family schedules. It's likely that your family has eating habits formed over many years, if not several generations.

When a family member suddenly decides to change the routine in any way, it's natural for some or all to resist the initiative. But, if your family and friends are not fully supportive and willing to compromise their own routines for your sake, then your challenge will be more difficult.

The best way to enlist support is to emphasize the positive health benefits of the Diet. After all, the resistance has more to do with disrupting comfortable routines than with your healthy objectives. If you can convince them that the change is not only good for you, but also for your family and friends, then it's more likely that they will support you. There's also a good chance that the benefits of healthy eating will be so obvious that everyone will want in on your newfound energy. This has been a way of life in the Gracie family for three generations. What's worked so well in our family can also work in yours.

5. What is most difficult for you in managing your weight?
For many people, two erroneous beliefs are at the heart of their inability to manage body weight. The first fallacy is that you can't control your weight…that you just can't win because it's all too complex, powerful, and overwhelming. This is something we also see in beginning jiu-jitsu students. If faced with an opponent who's bigger and stronger, they're convinced they're going to get beat up even before anything happens. They don't understand that the whole point of

jiu-jitsu is to empower the weak against the strong, based on information, efficiency, and confidence. So the initial principle a student needs to grasp is trust in the system. Trust that it really is possible to defend against a seemingly formidable adversary. And remember: That adversary is not chocolate or fried chicken or mashed potatoes. The real opponent is the enemy within – your belief that you can't change and you can't achieve your goals. So, you've got to defend yourself from yourself by developing confidence in the program.

The second misconception is that you're more tired than you actually are. This mindset holds people back at the very moment when real progress is just becoming possible. It sets in when you hit the inevitable plateau where the novelty of a new behavior is gone and fruits of the labor have yet to appear. Prepare for this by knowing that the high of beginning a new lifestyle is a delightful, but short-term feeling. One morning you're going to wake up and say, "Keeping track of these food groups is too much trouble," or, "I'm not losing weight fast enough." If you're expecting the plateau, you'll be better prepared to remain committed to the regimen and achieve your goals. If you succumb to the letdown and quit the Diet, you will have allowed the enemy within to win the round. It's not the end of the world, just start again. Remember, this match has no time limits – it's for the rest of your life!

6. What can you do to make following the Diet easy and enjoyable?
You're already taking the first step by answering these questions and establishing a base point from which to start. Record your answers so that when you reassess your progress in a few weeks, you will appreciate the changes in your eating habits. Of course, you will already feel the difference,

but seeing your progress on paper helps you to really appreciate your accomplishment.

7. What was your body weight at each of the following ages?
- 15/20   - 20/30   - 30/40   - 40/present

8. What do you believe would be your ideal weight at this time?

9. Have you followed any other diets for an extended period of time? Which one?

10. How long did you stick with the diets?

11. What were your results?

12. What were the positives and negatives of the diets you followed?

13. Why did you stop?

14. What did you learn from these programs regarding your weight?

15. Why do you want to begin the Gracie Diet now?

16. Which meals do you regularly eat?
- Breakfast
- Brunch
- Lunch
- Dinner

17. When do you snack?
- Morning
- Afternoon
- Evening
- Late at night
- Throughout the day

18. What are your favorite snack foods?

19. How often do you eat in restaurants or order food delivered?

20. How many times each day do you eat the following foods?
- Starch (bread, cereal, pasta, rice, potato)
- Fruits
- Vegetables
- Dairy (milk, yogurt)
- Meat, fish, poultry
- Fat (butter, margarine, mayonnaise, oil, salad dressing)
- Sweets (candy, cake, regular soda, juice)

21. How much of these beverages do you drink daily?
- Water
- Coffee
- Tea
- Soda
- Juice
- Alcohol

22. What are the most difficult times of the day for you to stay within a diet?
- Morning

- Afternoon
- Early Evening
- Late Evening
- All Day

23. What do you see as your major food temptations?
- Sweets – candy, cookies, cakes, sodas
- Starches – breads, potatoes, pasta, chips
- Butter
- Meats

24. During holidays or when eating in a restaurant, do you:
- Eat whatever you want to enjoy?
- Eat whatever you want and then eat more carefully for the next few days?
- Stick with your diet plan in these situations?

25. How frequently do you eat in each of these environments?
- While working, at your desk, or elsewhere
- With friends and/or family
- Alone
- In front of the television

26. How often are your meals:
- Home cooked
- Fast food
- A mix of fast food and home cooked
- Only healthy foods
- Restaurant / take out or delivery

27. Pick your favorite part of a restaurant meal:
- Bread / Chips

- Appetizers
- Salad
- Main Course
- Dessert

28. How often do you take second portions?
- Never
- Occasionally
- Almost always

29. How often do you eat meat?
- Never
- Occasionally
- Quite often

30. Do you have any health problems? For how long?
- Gastrointestinal (heartburn, IBS, esophagitis, etc.) _____
- High blood pressure _____
- High cholesterol _____
- Diabetes _____
- Excess weight _____
- Other _____

Now that you have a base point for your current eating habits, you're ready to take action. In the next chapter, we'll discuss the hardest part of the Diet – forming healthy eating habits. No worries though, I will show you the formula for success!

Having the Willpower to Resist Temptation… And Feel Good About It Afterwards

Following this program has positive benefits way beyond improving your health. Surprising as it may seem, the sense of responsibility and personal discipline that I've found in following these eating guidelines have been the real foundation of my training in jiu-jitsu, not the other way around. My ability to resist social pressures and to do the right thing for my health has set an example for my family and friends with far-reaching, long-lasting effects. Through the Gracie Diet, you will learn that the purpose of a meal is to nourish your body, not fill your belly. You will learn to control your impulses, and once you can do that, anything is possible.

Points to Remember:
- The Gracie Diet is more than a list of food combinations. It's the beginning of a new and healthier way of life.
- Your motivation to be healthy will overcome any limitations posed by your current physical condition.
- Never let yourself think that change is beyond your control. Not only do you have the power to defeat the enemy within, but you can start today!

 The Gracie Diet In A Nutshell

- Your motivation and success will increase as you realize that you're not doing it only for yourself.
- Digestion starts in your mouth. Chew your foods well, and slowly drink your juices, allowing plenty of time to salivate.
- The best way to help your children develop a healthy lifestyle is by setting a good example.

CHAPTER 4:

"Your fight is against yourself, not with anyone else. It is you that you must overcome, in other words, your flaws, your vices, your desires, your thoughts, etc…The only thing to fear, is the enemy within."

- André Luiz

The Hard Part: Changing Your Eating Habits

The key to good health is to consume foods in a way that ensures efficient digestion and maximizes nutritional benefits, while keeping the body alkaline. A watermelon is a watermelon, but how you eat it makes a difference in how well it serves your body. I'm suggesting that you make a meal of watermelon by eating it with toast or a tapioca tortilla with fresh, mild white cheese, and honey, instead of eating it as a dessert after a cooked meal. I'll try to answer all of your questions about the concept of food combinations in the next few pages. When you finish reading this chapter, you will have a new perspective on how to eat.

It is important to keep an open mind during this phase. Remember this investment in your health is priceless. You can be the richest person in the land, but without good health, you can't enjoy the fruits of your labor in your golden years. Imagine yourself with a major illness that prevents you from playing with your children or grandchildren, enjoying a walk on a sandy beach, admiring a sunset, or having the physical stamina to travel around the world. We all know people who have worked hard all of their lives to acquire a fortune, only to spend it on drugs, healthcare, and surgeries in a desperate battle to regain the health they mortgaged through bad eating habits in their youth. That is not what you want. The good news is that it's never too late, and the sooner you start the more likely you'll preserve your health as you age.

Once you start, the immediate changes in your well-being will motivate you to continue making healthy choices, creating a cycle of infinite possibilities. It's difficult to break lifelong habits and re-educate your body, so anticipate some slips as part of the process. Your ability to rise after falling takes strength and perseverance. You have nothing to lose and everything to gain. After all, in a few weeks, if you really think this is not a good program for you, just go back to your old ways.

The Belt Graduation System
A new student begins martial arts training as a white belt, then progresses through the ranks until achieving a black belt indicating mastery of the art. I've developed a similar system for tracking and motivating your transition from beginner to mastery of the Gracie Diet. Each rank requires learning and applying selected principles before moving to the next level of difficulty. Let's get started!

White belt
1- **Drink a glass of water when you awaken.** During the night, our body loses water through breathing, sweating, or going to the bathroom, so we awaken feeling thirsty and "dried up." Kick start your system with a glass of water first thing in the morning.
Observation: After drinking the water, leave the empty glass on the table next your bed to remind you to refill it for the next morning and help you develop the new habit.
2- **Wash your hands before every meal.** The transmission of harmful germs by hand contact is a constant health concern.
Observation: Use soap and water.

3- During the first week, record what you eat or drink, and the time of consumption. This will keep you accountable, and serve as a great comparative reference when you reflect on the experience in a few weeks.
Observation: Use the calendar on pages 56-57 and include as much detail as you can.

Blue belt
1- Continue the white belt habits.
Observation: Discontinue recording meals (unless you want to extend the record keeping for personal use).
2- **Gradually eliminate desserts after cooked meals.** If you eat dessert, sweets, or fruits every day, then start doing it every other day, and then every second day, and third day, and so on, until you break the habit.
Observation: When you finish your meal, you should not be hungry. Dessert is all about taste, and the price you will pay for it in the long run is not worth it!
3- **Eliminate all sodas.** Sodas are loaded with sugar and are proven to increase the risk of diabetes, heart diseases, obesity, etc.
Observation: With cooked foods, drink water, carbonated water, fresh coconut water, fresh vegetable juices, or teas without lemon or sugar.

Purple belt
1- Continue the blue belt habits.
2- **Start following the combinations of the Gracie Diet Table.** The table is on page 80-82.
Observation: Place a copy on your refrigerator.
3- **Eliminate pork and derivatives.** Undercooked pork was once a major cause of a parasitic disease called trichinosis, therefore we have eliminated it from our regimen.

Observation: A World Health Organization study determined that processed pork meat such as bacon, hot dogs, and sausage, cause cancer. The WHO also reported that red meat, pork, and lamb are probably cancer-causing foods as well.

Brown belt
1- Carry on the purple belt habits.
2- **Space meals at least 4 1/2 hours apart.** It is crucial that a meal is completely digested before you add more food to your stomach.
Observation: Do not snack between meals, but you may drink water.
3- **Eat right six days a week.** The seventh day is a cheat day! Eat and drink whatever you want. If you combine your foods properly and space your meals correctly for six days, your body will reject unhealthy eating habits! The queasiness you will feel should bring you to your senses, and motivate you to eat right every day.
Observation: When your body is working perfectly, you will more easily sense imbalance, identify the cause of the problem, and you'll know how to fix it!

Black belt
1- Carry on the brown belt habits.
2- **Eat right every day.** You will not only have abundant energy and will feel great, but also everyone will notice the difference.
Observation: If you choose to relax the diet discipline for a special occasion, don't worry about it because now you are in charge of your health!
3 Share the knowledge.
Observation: By sharing the benefits of your new eating habits, your level of conviction and understanding of the program will increase and inspire you to stay on the right path.

NOTE:
You should change belts levels within two weeks. If you are already following some of the rules, like washing your hands before a meal or not drinking sodas, then simply start drinking a glass of water and eliminating desserts. Congratulations! You're already a blue belt!

Your Current Eating Habits
Let's define your starting point by writing down your current eating habits. Use the following chart to record everything you eat and drink for one week. Document every detail – meal times, types of salad dressings, drinks, snacks, desserts, bread types, and how full you feel after each meal. Use the vertical column as a gas tank gauge and treat each box as 20% of your tank. Be sure to record your starting weight and consider taking a photograph to document your appearance before the diet. Record your answers in the book, or on a separate sheet of paper.

List Your Current Eating Habits

	BREAKFAST	SNACK	LUNCH
MON	TIME:	TIME:	TIME:
TUE	TIME:	TIME:	TIME:
WED	TIME:	TIME:	TIME:
THUR	TIME:	TIME:	TIME:
FRI	TIME:	TIME:	TIME:
SAT	TIME:	TIME:	TIME:
SUN	TIME:	TIME:	TIME:

Be As Detailed As Possible

SNACK	DINNER	SNACK
TIME:	TIME:	TIME:
TIME:	TIME:	TIME:
TIME:	TIME:	TIME:
TIME:	TIME:	TIME:
TIME:	TIME:	TIME:
TIME:	TIME:	TIME:
TIME:	TIME:	TIME:

Once you integrate the belt system into your eating routine, you'll appreciate the program's simplicity. You will feel the benefits of healthy eating before your first promotion. I have prepared a 14-day menu (page 132-135) to help you in the first few weeks of the program since some find the food combinations to be intimidating. Or, you can go directly to the full Gracie Diet Table of Combinations in Chapter 7 and create your own combinations.

You're on your way to achieving the well-being your body deserves. Remember, sooner or later you'll discover that your health is indeed the single most important thing in your life!

Your First Meal the Gracie Way
Your first meal should be a well-planned positive experience, that inspires you to want to repeat it. I recommend you try a sweet fruit-based (Group C) meal. Try sharing this meal with a friend or a loved one. If you have children, I recommend that you bring them in for this because it's a great opportunity to plant a seed in their heads. Let them experience a sweet meal that is natural and healthier than candy bars and a soda. If they enjoy the fruit meal, ask them if they would like to repeat it once a week. There is a good chance they will like it indeed, and then it will be easier to try another meal. Educating someone on how to make healthy choices is the best present you can give them, especially your children. They will appreciate and respect you for that. From this point on, you will take control, not only of your health through the purpose and awareness of everything you eat, but more importantly, you will develop a discipline that will increase your self-esteem and that will create endless possibilities! Eat to live, don't live to eat!

THREE SUGGESTIONS:

1) Pears, cottage cheese, and honey.

Selection: There are acidic and there are sweet pears. Make sure you use the sweet kind (D'anjou, Comice, etc.) They should look nice (no bruises), and will probably not be ripe, so you may have to wait a few days for them to be ready.

Preparation: Whenever they are ripe (soft to the touch), and it's mealtime, you should wash and peel them. Cut them into pieces, put them into a bowl with a spoon of cottage cheese and pour some honey over. Serving: 2-3 pears per person.

Equipment: A peeler or a knife.

2) Dates or honey, and fresh white cheese or fresh coconut meat, with crackers and watermelon juice.

Selection: Choose a ripe watermelon, some rye or whole wheat crackers (not both together), fresh cheese or fresh coconut meat, and Madjool dates. Chill the watermelon so that it is cold at meal time.

Preparation: Place 6-8 dates onto a bowl with warm water for 60 seconds to loosen the skin. Then gently remove the skin. Use the tip of a knife to remove the seed. Spread the fresh cheese (or a scoop of coconut meat) on the crackers and place the prepared dates or honey on top. (Video tutorial available at www.GracieDiet.com). Next, wash the watermelon, and fill the blender halfway with chunks small enough to blend without adding water. Blend for 20-30 seconds, then strain the liquid through a Gracie Juice Bag into a bowl (Video tutorial available at www.GracieDiet.com). Serving: 1-2 people.

Equipment: A blender, a Gracie Juice Bag, a bowl, and a knife.

3) Apple juice, bananas, and cream cheese smoothie.
Selection: Use sweet apples (red delicious, Gala, Fuji) and ripe bananas.
Preparation: Wash, peel, and slice four apples. Feed the apple slices through the juicer. Pour the juice into a blender. Add 4-5 bananas and a teaspoon of cream cheese or fresh coconut meat (optional) and blend it for 30-60 seconds. (Video tutorial available at www.GracieDiet.com)
Servings: 1-2 people.
Equipment: A juicer, a blender, and a peeler or a knife.

Doesn't it take a lot of time and work to prepare these meals?
For breakfast, at least three or four days a week, I prepare a smoothie made from bananas blended with a freshly squeezed fruit juice of watermelon, cantaloupe, or red delicious apples, plus a teaspoon of cream cheese or better yet, fresh coconut meat. Peeling five bananas and putting them in the blender takes less than one minute. The process of washing, cutting, and juicing a cantaloupe can also be done in less than five minutes (We use the Champion Juicer – www.GracieDiet.com). Scooping the meat out of a fresh coconut takes one minute. Blending the ingredients takes less than one minute, and the clean-up takes about five minutes. So, there you have it – a delicious and healthy breakfast prepared in about 12 minutes. I guarantee that you will feel a lot better than if you had a bowl of cereal with milk, a glass of grapefruit juice, and a cup of coffee.

Points to Remember:
- Don't feel that you must immediately change all your eating habits. Use the Belt Graduation System to guide and motivate you.
- It is very important that you start planning your meals, instead of just eating whatever is available.
- Choose breads made from one kind of grain: wheat, rye, etc. (Group B).

 The Gracie Diet In A Nutshell

- To juice apples, melons, pineapple, carrots, etc., use a juicer.
- For watermelon or grape juices, use a blender. After blending, strain the juice through a juice bag into a bowl.
- Prepare the juices for immediate consumption. The nutritional value of juices start diminishing as soon as they are made.

CHAPTER 5:

"People are fed by a food industry, which pays no attention to health, and are treated by a health industry, which pays no attention to food."

- Wendell Berry

Getting Started
It is natural to justify bad behavior to diminish our sense of guilt for having made a poor choice. The classical example is the cigarette. The smoker knows smoking is harmful, but can't or chooses not to stop despite the negative consequences that will result from the activity. We know that smoking is harmful. That is why many countries ban cigarette advertisements, require health risk warnings on packages, and prohibit smoking in public spaces.

Consuming unhealthy food can be as harmful as smoking. But, we allow the food industry to mislead consumers with packaging that promotes pleasure and convenience. The attack on your health is subtle. The food industry, led by fast food chains, and soda manufacturers, lures customers to their products at a young age and creates a life-long addiction to the brand in search of financial profit. They're not just taking your money; they are taking your life!

After years of bombardment by hormones, trans fat, sugar, GMOs, and countless chemical additives, your body will reflect the inevitable consequences of poor eating habits. You'll find yourself taking medicine for obesity, diabetes, heart problems, high blood pressure, gastrointestinal issues, and more. If that's not enough, the medicines themselves may cause side effects more dangerous than the problems they were supposed to treat. Just listen to the disclaimers that follow every television commercial for wonder drugs! It seems like a sinister plot to create lifelong dependency to the multi-billion dollar pharmaceutical industry. The food industry and the labs have set up a circus, and want you to be the clown.

Make healthy eating into a habit
Your health is the most important thing in your life. In the Gracie family, we take this matter very seriously and believe that refueling your body with healthy food is perhaps the single most important part of your daily routine. A meal at our house is almost ceremonial. It starts with the food selection.

As a boy in Brazil, I watched my father and my uncle buy fruits at the central produce market every week. They fussed over every selection to ensure that we not only had the right foods, but also that they were fresh, ripe, and tasty so that, as children, we would learn to like healthy food. I adopted the same ritual. For the last 35 years, once a week at dawn, rain or shine, I've been going to the Wholesale Central Produce Market, in downtown Los Angeles, to buy crates of fruits.

The ability to break old eating habits and develop new ones is the basis for succeeding at any diet. When you can decline your favorite dish because you know it's not good for you; or choose a glass of water over a snack because you know it's not time to eat; or stop eating when you're 80% full because you know that you're sufficiently nourished, you will find that you've developed willpower and control that will carry over to all aspects of your life. The ability to master your impulses is highly rewarding, and demonstrates a winner's attitude. The time has come for you to experiment with this!

This reeducation process is like learning a new skill – like sewing, playing the piano, bowling, or flying a helicopter. You must follow a plan, which includes getting quality instruction, buying the necessary equipment, and committing to it. It doesn't matter how much time goes by, if we have fond memories of a fun and positive hobby or activity from our past, the thought of it will always bring us joy. Many times these very activities, or even our memories of them, serve as motivators as we age. So stick with the Diet – it could become the most pleasant and rewarding experience of your life. After all, if you want to enjoy better health in ten years, then start now!

Changing Habits Requires a Plan
After all the years that I've been helping people to improve their eating habits, I've learned one very important fact: If people fail, it's usually because they failed to plan. Make the time to study and understand the program, so that you are less likely to get confused, make mistakes, get frustrated, and give up. Otherwise, you may become discouraged, revert to old eating habits, and accept the physical and psychological consequences of a lost battle. That won't help your self-esteem. Often, you don't feel the chains of habit until they are too strong to break. Basic behaviors just don't change by themselves.

The key to forming new habits is to start with small changes. For example, try to brush your teeth with your weak hand for seven days. At first, you find yourself forgetting to make the change because your brushing habits have become such a deeply ingrained reflex. However, if you store your toothbrush on the opposite side of the sink, this will influence your habit-forming awareness, and help create a framework for a new way of thinking about food.

Likewise, you can ease into the Gracie Diet by making simple changes to your eating habits. The Belt Graduation System will help. Again, my objective is to show you that regardless of your current eating habits, there is a way for you to improve them. Sometimes, all you need to do is to avoid one simple ingredient, and you can prevent harmful consequences. Remember, too, that you will not deprive yourself from the pleasure of eating. This is absolutely not a restrictive diet like so many that strictly limit quantities only to have participants counting the days until they can return to their old habits. We're talking about a new lifestyle that allows you to eat virtually anything, as long as you follow the combination guidelines, while giving you abundant energy, eliminating excess weight, and preventing a variety of common diet-related health problems.

People are so accustomed to feeling good one day and bad on the other, that they assume it's normal. It is not! Your body is an amazingly efficient machine. A headache, heartburn, or a few extra pounds, clearly indicate that the machine is not working as it should. We must heed these indications and adjust our eating habits, so that the body can operate as designed – perfectly!

Reviewing the Basic Concepts

A – Never eat dessert.
Whenever you eat cooked food prepared with fat, oil, or butter you may eat until you're 80% full. However, avoid consuming sugar, sweets, juices, or fruits with this meal. In other words, never eat dessert.

B – One starch per meal.
Instead of eating a hamburger with bun (wheat) and fries (potatoes), eat two hamburgers and no fries, or the meat patties (without the buns) and all the fries you want. Be especially attentive when you go to a restaurant and the

waiter drops that basket with warm bread on your table. If you want to eat the bread (wheat) while they prepare your food, then you should order pasta, pizza, or a sandwich prepared from the same starch as the bread (wheat). Avoid anything derived from another starch, like risotto (rice) or fries (potatoes). They may taste good, but in combination with another starch, they are not good for you.

C- Allow for at least 4 ½ hours between meals.
One diet theory contends that eating several small meals throughout the day forces the digestive system to work constantly and, as a result, burns more calories and increases weight loss. Another argues that eating numerous small meals helps stave hunger and prevents overeating. The Gracie Diet rejects both theories. Frequent eating prevents complete digestion and causes fermentation and acidity. The body needs at least 4 ½ hours (4 hours for children) between meals to complete this process. I promise you will not starve, and you will feel much better. The healthiest way to control hunger is to drink water or fresh coconut water between meals. Don't snack!

D – Eliminate sodas.
Here's what you get in typical can of soda:
Sugar: Ten teaspoons of low-quality sugar will negatively affect your cholesterol, insulin, and blood pressure while promoting health problems such as cardiac disease, diabetes, and obesity. Diet sodas are even worse, since they contain aspartame which has been linked to an additional set of health issues such as sugar addiction, emotional diseases, weight gain, cancer, and leukemia.
Phosphoric acid: Affects the body's capacity to absorb calcium leading to weakened bones and teeth, and osteoporosis.

Caffeine: Drinks that contain caffeine increase cholesterol and blood pressure, increase heart rate, and may contribute to lumps in breasts, birth defects, and cancer.

High fructose corn syrup: The food industry uses this sweetener, produced from GMO corn, in a countless number of products. It's linked to obesity, heart diseases, diabetes, and high blood pressure.

Caramel coloring: The National Toxicity Program found "clear evidence" of the toxicity of caramel coloring (4-MEI) in sodas, and connected it to infertility, thyroid dysfunction, liver and lung cancer.[5]

I am often told that following these basic concepts of the Gracie Diet deprives me from enjoying some of the greatest pleasures of eating. I never believed that because I have always enjoyed eating. More importantly, I have remained healthy and cavity-free for over 65 years as a result of observing these rules!

Aren't all these fresh fruits and vegetables very expensive?
I believe that money spent on natural foods today is money saved on medical bills tomorrow. You would be amazed at how much money you spend for snack foods, candy, or coffee with a pastry. Apply that money toward healthy foods and I think you'll find your food budget has increased very little, if at all. More important, you'll feel good all of the time – and that is priceless.

---

[5] http://www.seattleorganicrestaurants.com/vegan-whole-food/Pepsi-Coca-Cola-harmful-ingredients.php

Points to Remember:
- Allow at least 4 ½ hours between meals. Don't snack!
- Never eat dessert or drink sodas.
- Do not mix different starches within the same meal.

 The Gracie Diet In A Nutshell

- Many breads or cereals (Group B) contain honey and/or fruits (Group C), or even more than one starch, therefore they do not combine with meats or vegetables (Group A) or milk (Group F). Read the labels.
- Consume your legumes and vegetables raw, or lightly sautéed, with garlic and onion, in olive oil or butter.
- The healthiest way to cook your legumes and vegetables is in a steamer to minimize the loss of nutrients.

PART TWO:

Using the Gracie Diet

CHAPTER 6:

"Few things are harder to put up with than the annoyance of a good example."
- Mark Twain

A Family Affair

Throughout this book, I've cited my childhood experiences as one of the most important factors in forming my own eating habits. The examples set by my relatives have stayed with me all of my life and I am now passing these habits to my children. Often, we only recognize and appreciate good habits once we're adults. Children almost always follow their hearts and their stomachs before they follow their heads... and both are organs without reasoning capabilities, so they don't always point in the right direction! My siblings and I were fortunate to not only have good examples set for us, but also to have parents who were so committed to our health that they trained us to eat properly by feeding us healthy food and not allowing us to eat that which was not. The most powerful tool of all was their personal example. In fact, example isn't the best way to educate, it's the only way. With that in mind, I encourage you to eat well not only for your own health, but also to set an example for your children and put them on the road to good health.

The Power of Example

The Gracie Diet is easy for me to follow because it's all I've ever known. There were no sodas, chocolate chip cookies, or candy bars to be found anywhere in the house...period. We ate when it was time to eat and if we got hungry before mealtime, a glass of water solved the problem. If not, we drank another one. No one ever starved to death. As a parent, I applied the same rules with my children and achieved the same positive results – children who, from birth, knew how and when to eat nutritious, healthy foods. I recognize your situation may be very different from mine.

I have heard many stories about the challenges families face when starting the Gracie way of eating. At first, everyone will be curious and want to try the meals – especially the fruit meals and smoothies. Their enthusiasm then quickly fades at the prospect of buying a juicer, keeping fresh fruit on hand, tracking food combinations, or modifying meal times. Don't let the waning interest dissuade you. Remember our discussion about the difficulty of breaking deeply ingrained habits and that you can't force a person to change their ways. They must decide on their own if the potential payoff is worth the sacrifice. The difficult part is accepting that you will be improving your health while your other family members will continue ruining theirs. The more aware you become, the more painful it is to ignore them.

It is very important to realize that your loved ones may not share your motivation to change your eating habits. I know of many cases in which one person in a household embraces the Gracie Diet, but starts World War III when they attempt to force the new rules on the rest of the family! You can't win without patience and consideration. Try doing all of the preparatory work yourself. Start by preparing the "Nectar of the Champions"— fresh melon juice, blended with bananas and açaí – and then bring to your companion while they're still in bed! Not only the delicious taste of a healthy breakfast, but the convenience of breakfast in bed, will create a positive experience that encourages your partner to try the routine. Do this for a few days and see if your companion will join you in embracing the new health concept.

The youngest ones should make the transition with ease

(if you and your spouse work together). For the first six months, feed your infant nothing but breast milk. Usually infants will eat every three hours. Then, you should introduce mashed fruits like bananas or sweet apple scraped with a spoon once a day (make sure the fruits are ripe and sweet tasting). Soon thereafter, you can add a meal of mashed vegetables, soups, etc. to the daily routine. Avoid acidic (Group D) fruit meals for youngsters. As you introduce heavier foods, the child will naturally be able to wait a little longer in between meals. Eventually, the goal is to get the child on a comfortable routine of eating Gracie Diet compliant meals every four hours.

A Quick and Simple Way to Kick the Junk Food Habit
Kids only think about taste — because it provides instant gratification. They simply don't care about long-term, harmful consequences. When you cut out the junk food, you have to fill the "junk food void" with an explanation. Keep it simple and honest. Tell them that you are going to cut down the junk food because it is not good for them. Then, get all of it out of the house and never bring it back in! The key element for this to work is that there can be no candy in the house, sodas in the refrigerator, or ice cream in the freezer. That means for everyone in the household. As you implement this new rule, expect a certain level of discontent from the troops. Do not feel sorry or get confused if you see tears or tantrums. Instead, take a deep breath and be fascinated by their dependency on junk food. Realize the seriousness of the situation and use it as a motivator to help you focus on your child's well-being. They will thank you later if they are kept out of the statistics on diabetes or the ever-growing number of obese children. Young children may have acquired a taste for "junk food" but at least they can't drive to

the store. They will only have access to it if you bring it home. Don't do it anymore. If you know it is not good for them, why would you?

What to Do When Kids Demand Junk Food

You must be patient and understand that they may go through withdrawals, just like a drug addict. In order to deal with that, you may want to have some sugarless gum stashed away for an emergency. With the older kids, you will need a different strategy. It is not wise to force them into it. There is a risk of rebellion because they may not have the understanding of the healthy-versus-unhealthy mindset. Furthermore, they have access to everything at school or at the local store. The best approach is communication and patience. Remind them that the saying is "An apple a day…" not, "A Hershey bar a day…" – and that eating junk food will have negative consequences in the future.

The Ultimate Halloween Trick

Halloween is a fun holiday filled with cool costumes, cool social events, and lots of candy. In the Gracie household, we use it as an opportunity to teach discipline and willpower. When the kids come home with their bags full of goodies, we pour the contents on the carpet and we separate everything into categories based on the type of treat. We let the kids keep a few pieces of gum and maybe one or two lollipops, with the understanding that the rest is not good for them and must go into the trash. I praise the kids for being strong enough to collect so much candy and not eat it, and I remind them that their remarkable self-control will pay dividends in the long run.

Birthdays and other parties

For young kids, attending a party seems like a weekly event between birthdays and school, club, team, and church functions. These events often offer cookies, snacks, and drinks as refreshments. In our family, we see these events as opportunities to teach our kids to make the right choices and practice discipline. You can help them by feeding them before the party. If possible, feed your child at home before they go to the party to reinforce the proper food combinations and the quality of their food. And, of course, it's easier to decline junk food on a full tummy. The other option is to allow them to eat at the party, but with you there to guide them through the proper choices and combinations. Ignore those who try to justify feeding your child unhealthy food by stating, "it's just a small piece" or "grandma made this specially for him." In time, your kids will learn to make their own selection. Remember to praise their strength of will, and to remind them that this attitude will ultimately benefits all aspects of their lives.

How to Win the Kids Over, One Bite at a Time

Eating is near the top of the list of pleasures. As you learn to prepare your meals the Gracie way, I am sure you will win over other family members, one bite at a time! Always encourage everyone else to try it. Whenever my kids brought friends over, I made sure they tried a fruit meal from the Gracie Diet. They loved it – and I would use those opportunities to explain the general concept of the Diet to our guests, in order to teach my own children. The surprise and curiosity on the guests' faces reminded my kids that they were eating something out of the ordinary, something special. It raised their level of consciousness about healthy eating. Gradually, as my children learned the concepts, they grew comfortable enough to do the explaining themselves.

If all of the above fails, then try for a partial conversion to the Diet. Consider, for example, reducing junk food consumption for one week to once every-other day instead of daily. Then, try to cut out junk food every-other two days for the second week, and so on. Maybe even say something like: "Let's see how much we save on candy bars and sodas for a month and use the money for a new video game, or a new outfit, instead."

What easy items can a parent prepare for their child's lunch?
Dates and cream cheese on pita or sourdough bread, or raisin bread and Monterey Jack cheese sandwich, with cantaloupe pieces and a bottle of water. Send it in a small lunch box with an ice pack. Alternate that with a couple of bananas and a red sweet apple. In time, as they learn about the combinations it will be OK for the kids to eat at the cafeteria. Remind them to stay away from the sauces. Be sure to talk with them and guide them on the process by explaining the importance and benefits of good health.

Points to Remember:
- Whenever possible, choose organic foods with minimum processing. It will pay off in the long run.
- Until you learn which group a certain food belongs to, you may need to check the Table of Foods in the book.
- Avoid fried foods.

The Gracie Diet In A Nutshell

- The Gracie Diet has worked for thousands of people and will work for you.
- Take deep breaths of clean air a few of times throughout the day.
- Try the diet – you have nothing to lose and everything to gain.

CHAPTER 7:

"Nobody ever did, or ever will, escape the consequences of his choices."

- Alfred A. Montapert

Don't Be Afraid to Ask for the Best

Our family prepares our meals at home where we can guarantee the quality, sanitation, and proper preparation of our food. To put it bluntly, I'm uncomfortable having strangers prepare my meals for me, especially since I have worked in a restaurant and am familiar with the many opportunities to cut corners on quality and sanitation. Nevertheless, you may have no choice but to eat out, so it's important that we address your options.

The first step is to ensure that you are eating high-quality food. The sooner you become selective about the quality of the food you eat, the better for you. Regardless of quality, you will feel better if you properly combine foods. In fact, properly combining lower-quality foods is better for you than improperly combining high-quality foods. But, properly combining high-quality foods is the best of all options. Good food is that which is organically grown free of pesticides, genetic modifications, preservatives, artificial flavorings, and other additives. Bad food is everything else.

Let's consider two types of chicken and cheese sandwiches. You could have a sandwich made with a free-ranging chicken that spent its days pecking and smiling until it naturally reached an ideal weight before finding its way to your lunch plate. Or, you could make a meal of the chicken that was quickly fattened by force-feeding loads of hormones while it spent its mercifully short life trapped in a cage until it was ready for shipping to your local restaurant or supermarket. You could choose cheese produced from the milk of hormone-free cows that roam the vast pastures, drink unpolluted waters, and are loved by the farmer (who calls them by name and milks them by hand every day). Or, you could choose the cheese from the cows that were fed hormone-laden grain to produce mass volumes of milk to which the dairy added all kinds of chemicals and colorings. You could select bread made from high-quality whole grain, grown under the golden sun of beautiful plains, or the cheap bleached white bread loaded with chemicals. You could opt for organic lettuce in those fancy plastic cases with the roots intact to preserve freshness and a validation date stamped on the label, or you could choose the other kind.

Question the nutritional value of everything you consume. Why eat meat? It is a great source of protein, but some studies associate meat consumption with health problems. And, what about the ethical considerations? Some religions equate the killing of animals to murder! What about milk as a source of calcium? Isn't cow milk meant for calves? Should we eat butter? Is margarine better or worse? Some say we should not consume canola oil, and only use coconut oil. Gluten – is it good or bad for you? Should we stop eating bread – a vital staple in much of the world's diet since the dawn of civilization? Eggs were once condemned for contributing to high cholesterol. Now, some consider it to be one the most complete foods. You can find different answers to all of these questions just like you can find contradictory views on this diet. When all is said and done, listen to your body. Do your own research and let the results guide you in your food choices and eating habits. I'm confident your findings will reinforce your faith in the Gracie diet.

For now, let's focus on the basic combination principles.

Your Guide to Food Combinations

The following pages will introduce you to the food groups and food combining principles – the hallmark of the Gracie Diet. The key thing to understand is that the food combination guidelines are not based on taste, appearance, or biological classification, and may go against traditional ways of food combining. Our way of pairing the foods optimizes the digestive process and increases energy, health, and longevity. These combinations are the result of almost 70 years of empirical research which has shown incredible results to a variety of health problems, especially those related to the intestines, recently referred to as "the second brain." Imagine that the thousands of people around the world that endorse these food combination concepts are telling the truth; that their lives have indeed changed for the better; that they no longer suffer from heartburn, gastritis, migraine headaches, or IBS; and that their diabetes and weight are under control. Is that not enough for you to at least try it?

Don't let the Table of Combinations intimidate you. Later, I will provide lots of real life examples that will clarify the combination guidelines, as well as an easy-to-follow 14-day integration plan so that you can adopt the Gracie Diet with ease.

THE GRACIE DIET TABLE

GROUP A | Foods that combine with each other and one of Group B.

MEATS & SEAFOOD

Chicken	Fish Eggs	Red Meat
Crab	Lobster	Shellfish
Crawfish	Mussels	Shrimp
Eggs	Octopus	Squid
Fish	Oysters	Turkey

FATS & OILY FOODS

Avocados	Cocoa	Olive Oil
Almonds	Fats in General	Peanuts
Butter / Margarine	Hazelnuts	Pine Nuts
Brazilian Nuts	Melted Cheeses	Sesame Seeds
Cashews	Nuts in General	Walnuts
Coconut - Dried	Olives	Wheat Germ

VEGETABLES & GREENS

Artichokes	Cilantro	Okra
Arugula	Corn – Fresh	Onions
Asparagus	Cucumbers	Oregano
Basil	Eggplants	Parsley
Bay Leaves	Endive	Peas - Fresh
Beets - Red	Garlic	Pumpkin
Bell Peppers	Ginger	Radish
Broccoli	Green Beans	Spinach
Brussels Sprouts	Green Onions	Soy - Fresh
Butternut Squash	Hearts of Palm	Turnip
Cabbage	Kale	Tomatoes - Cooked
Carrots	Leeks	Watercress
Cauliflower	Lettuce	Zucchini
Celery	Mushrooms	

THE GRACIE DIET TABLE

GROUP B | *Starches do not combine with each other.*

Barley	Dry Peas	Quinoa
Breadfruit	Dry Soy	Rice
Cereals in General	Lentils	Rye
Chestnuts	Manioc	Sweet Potatoes
Dry Beans	Oats	Wheat and Derivatives
Dry Corn/Flour	Potatoes	Yams

GROUP C | *Foods that combine with each other and with one of Group B, if not prepared with fat.*

Apples* - Red	Guava*	Watermelon
Açaí	Honey	All Fresh Sweet Fruits
Bananas - Dried, Baked or Cooked	Jaca Fruit	
	Melons	Teas of Leaves or Peel of: Orange, Lemon, Apple, Fig Leaves, Black Tea, Mate, Cider, Chamomile, Various Herbs, etc.
Cherimoya*	Papaya	
Cheese - Fresh	Pears - Sweet	
Coconuts - Fresh	Persimmons	
Cottage Cheese	Plums* - Sweet	
Cream Cheese	Prunes	
Monterey Jack	Raisins	
Dates	Ricotta Cheese	
Figs - Fresh	Sugar Cane	
Grapes* - Sweet	Sugar in General	

*These are sub-acidic fruits and should not be eaten with each other.

THE GRACIE DIET TABLE

GROUP D	*Acidic Fruits* do not combine with each other or with anything else.

Apples - Green	Kiwis	Plums - Acidic
Apricots	Lemons	Pomegranate
Blackberries	Lime	Quince
Blueberries	Mangos	Raspberries
Cherries	Oranges	Strawberries
Currants	Peaches	Tangerines
Grapes - Acidic	Pears - Acidic	Tomatoes
Grapefruit	Pineapples	All Acidic Fruits

GROUP E	*Raw Bananas*

Combine With:		Do Not Combine With:	
Apples - Red	Papaya	Avocados	Sugar Cane Oil / Fat in General
Cheese - Fresh	Pears - Sweet	Dried Fruits	
Cream - Fresh	Watermelon	Honey	All of Group A or B
Grapes - Sweet	All Fresh Sweet Fruits	Oily Fruits	
Melons		Sugar in General	
Milk			

GROUP F	*Milk*

Combine With:		Do Not Combine With:	
Bananas - Raw or Baked	Milk Derivatives Except: Curdled Milk, Kefir, Yogurt, and Other Curdled Dairy Products, which should be eaten alone.	Avocados	Oily Fruits
Cooked Yolk		Egg Whites	Olives
Artificial Sweeteners		Fruits in General	Sugar in General
All of Group B		Meats in General	All of Group A
		Oils and Fats	

OBSERVATIONS:

Author's Note:
The original table of combinations which Uncle Carlos developed, included "Group G" which explained the proper combinations for "fresh milk cream," the kind we found on dairy farms in the old days. However, unless you have a cow in your backyard, it is virtually impossible to find the kind of fresh milk cream that he was referring to, since everything is processed before it is available to the public. Therefore, I decided to leave Group G out. Also, for the purpose of the Diet, you should treat the "milk cream" that you will find in stores as milk.

Gracie Diet Combination Summary
The Gracie Diet is very simple, but I realize that until you get some real life practice, the table of foods can be quite intimidating. Here's all you really need to know. Aside from an occasional meal that includes acidic fruits (Group D), raw bananas (Group E) or milk (Group F), each of which has their own very specific combination rules (see table to the left), almost all meals are either Group A-based or Group C-based. To keep things simple, at home we refer to our Group A meals as "cooked" meals, even though many of the foods in Group A are not actually cooked, and we refer to Group C meals as our "sweet" meals, even though not all foods in Group C are sweet. Just remember, in a Group A meal you can have any combination of the Group A foods together – vegetables, meats, fats, etc. – and one starch from Group B. In a Group C meal you can have any combination of the Group C foods together – sweet fruits, cheeses, etc. – as well as one starch from Group B, as long as you do not add fat (oil, butter, etc). Most importantly, never mix Group A with Group C.

Neutral Foods
Raw or cooked egg yolk, coconut water, brewer's yeast, coffee, and several kinds of tea are considered neutral and compatible with any food.

Coffee
Because the Gracie Diet enables your body to use less energy for digestion, you may find that the extra boost you once sought from caffeine is no longer necessary to start your day. If you enjoy coffee, you may still drink it with your meal. However, keep in mind that it is acidic, therefore, the less coffee you drink, the better. Remember to avoid sweetening your coffee with sugar as it does not combine with foods prepared with fat such as oil or butter. If necessary, use stevia or an artificial sweetener, but know that some of them may be harmful to your health.

Breads
Bread should be made from whole flour and should not be consumed within 24 hours of being baked. Then, prior to being eaten, it should be toasted or oven-warmed.

Avoid
Sweets, canned foods in syrup, pepper, clove, cinnamon, pickles, and vinegar.

Never Eat
Don't eat pork in any form.

Missing Foods
Although the Gracie Diet Table provides a comprehensive list of the foods found in Brazil when Carlos Gracie developed the Diet, you may find a favorite food that isn't on the list. If so, categorize the food by placing in the group with similar characteristics and

apply that group's combination guidelines. You can also ask questions at www.GracieDiet.com or on my Facebook page at Rorion Gracie.

Points to Remember:
- Avocado is a great substitute for meats and fish, since it is a good source of protein and free of toxins.
- Do not overeat cheeses. Choose fresh, mild cheeses like cottage or ricotta, instead of aged or spicy cheese like Roquefort, Camembert, or pepper-flavored ones.
- Cheeses belong to Group C, however, when melted they move to Group A.

 The Gracie Diet In A Nutshell

- Whenever you eat cooked foods (Group A) you may add raw cashews, Brazil nuts, walnuts, Macadamia nuts, or avocados as a source of protein.
- Salads are very healthy. For even greater benefits from legumes and vegetables, juice them. Start with carrots, and then add other foods from Group A.
- Eat lots of dark green leaves.

CHAPTER 8:

"A great amount of good can be done by enlightening all to whom we have access, as to the best means, not only of curing the sick, but preventing disease and suffering."

- Ellen G. White

How to Eat Healthily When You're on the Run

Knowing what to order when eating out can make a huge difference in your well-being. In this section, we'll see how to order from some popular restaurants and fast food chains. Note that I included this chapter to demonstrate how the Gracie Diet can accommodate familiar eating patterns and habits, not to endorse eating in restaurants. I have eaten in a few of these places and I know I am better off if I never repeat that mistake. However, if you have no choice, there are ways to order food that can make the meal less harmful. I will show you how to order and how to avoid the common mistakes that will make a big difference.

It can be difficult to order plain food. Ordering a salad with some pasta and a piece of fish seems simple enough. However, when they add the dressing to the salad, the sauce over the pasta, and a squeeze of lemon over your fish, it changes everything! That is enough to transform what could have been a harmless meal into something that is actually harmful to your health. You have options.

When away from home, go to the local supermarket and get some seasonal fruits, like a few ripe bananas and some red delicious apples or a slice of watermelon. If you know you're going to be out and about at mealtime, take your fruits with you. Plan ahead and you can't go wrong! If you don't have access to a market, then try to order food that you can "simplify." I rarely eat at fast food restaurants, but a few years ago during a long trip I stopped at a restaurant of a popular chain to use the restroom. Because it was way past my time to eat and I had no other options, I ordered a couple of fish filet sandwiches with no sauce, no pickles, and a glass of water. No matter where you are, there is always a way to improvise.

Another challenge you'll face in a restaurant is food quality. I'm not talking about taste or portion, but the freshness and purity of the food. Clearly, a restaurant exists to make a profit. Their balance sheet determines the quality of food they will use, and with rare exceptions, the quality will vary from bad to worse. From the kind of lettuce to the quality of the meat and the type of bread, everything is calculated to make it affordable to all and by doing so generate a bigger profit for them. Every month, approximately 9 out of 10 American children visit a McDonald's restaurant. In 1970, Americans spent about $6 billion on fast food. In 2015, that spending rose to $384 billion dollars.

The problem is that your health is not a priority in the cost-profit equation. Since nothing impacts your health like the food you eat, you can't ignore the fact that it is your responsibility to make the right choices. You must look out for your health and that of your loved ones, because nobody else will. Studies indicate that 7 out of 10 Americans opt for fast food at least three times a week, and that seven percent eat fast food everyday. Perhaps that is why the estimated health costs for 2025 will exceed five trillion dollars.

Learn the Food Selection Process

When ordering at a familiar restaurant, you probably know what you want. Based on your choice of entrée, you can build the rest of your meal. Follow this process:

Suppose you're considering a dish of fish, rice, and vegetables. That means you can't eat the wheat bread the waiter will bring to the table because it does not combine with rice (both are in Group B: Starches and therefore do not combine with one another). You could, however, eat the bread if you substitute the rice for pasta with the fish and vegetables, because the pasta and the bread are both made out of wheat (Group B). Just be sure to verify that there are no potatoes mixed in with the vegetables since they are a different starch (Group B) and do not combine with wheat either. If you order a salad, use no dressing other than olive oil and salt. Insist that all sauces or dressings are served on the side to help you to eat less while avoiding condiments that not only modify the taste of the food, but also contain unhealthy combinations of vinegar, pepper, lemon, and sugar.

Many appetizers are acceptable – Carpaccio, crab cakes, spinach artichoke dip, avocado egg rolls, etc. Once again, you must think about the meal as a whole, and be sure to ask what the spinach artichoke dip is served with. If it's served with bread, it means that it's OK with the pasta from the entrée since they are both made from the same starch – wheat (Group B). If it's served with corn or potato chips instead, since they are different starches, it would not combine. The same principle applies to egg rolls. The wrap is made with wheat, so you're OK if you've ordered pasta.

Learn to drink only water without lemon or lime. If you enjoy carbonation, then drink sparkling water instead of soda. Fresh coconut water is also a wise alternative. I often bring a coconut with me to the restaurant, and by the look on everyone's face, I know they all wish they had one too.

Once again, never eat dessert!

How Well Do You Know the Combinations?
This section will help determine your understanding of the Gracie Diet Table of food combining. Feel free to check the table as you analyze the options. In the following 10 sets find the one food that does not combine with all the others:

1.
a) Mashed potatoes
b) French fries
c) Rice
d) Baked potatoes
e) Turkey

2.
a) Eggs
b) Bread
c) Beef
d) Pasta
e) They all combine.

3.
a) Potato chips
b) Tuna sandwich
c) Pizza
d) Cheeseburger
e) Spaghetti

4.
a) Cantaloupe
b) Watermelon
c) Sweet pears
d) Blueberries
e) Bananas

5.
a) Honeydew melon
b) Persimmons
c) Green apples
d) Papaya
e) Honey

6.
a) Wheat bread
b) Watermelon juice
c) Guava jelly
d) Peanut butter
e) Monterey Jack cheese

7.
a) Bananas
b) Red apples
c) Cantaloupe
d) Kiwi
e) Papaya

8.
a) Pickles
b) Broccoli
c) Spinach
d) Cucumber
e) Potatoes

9.
a) Fish
b) Bacon
c) Chicken
d) Beef
e) Rice

10.
a) Sparkling water
b) Carrot juice
c) Coconut water
d) Coffee
e) They all combine.

In the next 10 sets, identify which meal violates the Gracie Diet combination guidelines.

11.
a) Rice, salmon, broccoli, cashews, carrot juice
b) Spaghetti, chicken, green beans, pizza, coconut water
c) Baked potatoes, French fries, lettuce, eggs
d) Beans, rice, turkey, squash, sparking water
e) They all combine.

12.
a) Watermelon juice, crackers, and Jack cheese
b) Cantaloupe juice, raisin bread, and cream cheese
c) Orange juice, wheat toast, and cottage cheese
d) Bananas, cream cheese, and red apples
e) They all combine.

13.

a) Cheeseburger, scrambled eggs, salad, and water
b) Pizza, avocado, chicken, sparkling water
c) Steak, rice, vegetables, coffee
d) Fish, spaghetti, green beans, lemonade
e) They all combine.

14.

a) Corn soup, grilled cheese sandwich, coconut water
b) Grilled chicken, pasta, avocado, fruit salad
c) Salmon, quinoa, broccoli, carrot juice
d) Sautéed vegetables, rice, beef, salad
e) They all combine.

15.

a) Peanut butter, jelly, bread, apple juice
b) Seafood risotto, squash, chamomile tea
c) Pizza, avocado, chicken, angel hair pasta, coffee
d) Black beans, green beans, walnuts, water
e) They all combine.

16.

a) Vegetables, rice, avocado, cashews, ice tea (no sugar)
b) Fish, spaghetti, carrots, broccoli, water
c) Chicken, pasta, salad, pistachios, sparkling water
d) Beef, mashed potatoes, celery, coconut water
e) They all combine.

17.

a) Rice, shrimp, vegetables, coconut water
b) Pizza, avocado, French fries, carrot juice
c) Baked potatoes, grilled halibut, asparagus, water

d) Pasta, chicken, salad, cashews, sparkling water
e) They all combine.

18.
a) Lettuce, cucumber, bell peppers, radish, vinegar
b) Spinach, heart of palm, cashews, olive oil, salt
c) Romaine lettuce, onions, olives, avocado, bell peppers
d) Arugula, broccoli, beets, celery, spinach
e) They all combine.

19.
a) Fish and chips
b) Macaroni and cheese
c) Hamburger and French fries
d) Bagels and coffee
e) They all combine.

20.
a) Cantaloupe, sweet pears, Monterey Jack cheese
b) Papaya, dates, cottage cheese
c) Honeydew melon, fresh figs, cream cheese
d) Watermelon, mangos, cottage cheese
e) Apples, bananas, cream cheese

Correct Answers:

1-c) Potatoes and Rice (Group B) are different starches and do not combine.
2-e) They all combine.
3-a) Wheat and Potatoes (Group B) are different starches and do not combine.
4-d) Blueberries (Group D) are acidic and do not combine with anything else.
5-c) Green apples (Group D) are acidic and do not combine with anything else.
6-d) Peanut butter (Group A) does not combine with fruits or sweets (Group C).
7-d) Kiwi (Group D) is acidic and should not be consumed with anything else.
8-a) Pickles are fermented cucumbers preserved in vinegar. They do not combine.
9-b) Bacon or any form of pork meat should never be consumed.
10-e) They all combine.
11-d) Beans and rice (Group B) are both starches and do not combine.
12-c) Orange juice (Group D) is acidic and does not combine with anything else.
13-d) Lemon (Group D) is acidic and does not combine with anything else.
14-b) Chicken and avocado (Group A) do not combine with fruits (Groups C or D).
15-a) Peanut butter (Group A) does not combine with sweets (Group C).
16-e) They all combine.
17-b) Pizza (wheat) and potatoes (Group B) are starches and do not combine.
18-a) Vinegar and all other spices do not combine and should be avoided.
19-c) The bun (wheat) and potatoes (Group B) are starches and don't combine.
20-d) Mango (Group D) is acidic and it should only be eaten by itself.

94 The Gracie Diet

Real Life Examples Drawn from the Menus of Popular Restaurants

Following are several samples of Group A meals from popular restaurants. A "NOTE" follows each of them suggesting the best way to order the dish to meet the combination requirements for the Gracie Diet. *WARNING: In many restaurants, the waiter will bring a basket of bread and butter to your table. Remember, the bread is made of wheat (Group B). So, you should only eat it if you plan on ordering an entrée that will combine with it.*

CHEESECAKE FACTORY

AVOCADO EGGROLLS

Avocado, sun-dried tomato, red onion, and cilantro deep fried in a crisp Chinese wrapper. Served with a dipping sauce.

NOTE: *Because the wrapper is made of wheat, you should plan on eating pasta as part of your entrée. Do not touch the sauce.*

MINI CRABCAKES

Louisiana crab served with mustard and tartar sauce.
NOTE: *Enjoy them without the mustard or tartar sauce.*

CHOPPED SALAD

Romaine lettuce, grilled chicken, tomato, avocado, corn, bacon, blue cheese, apple, and vinaigrette.
NOTE: *Ask for no tomatoes, bacon, blue cheese, apple slices, or vinaigrette.*

REMEMBER: *Drink water, sparkling water, or tea without lemon or sugar. And no dessert!*

LUAU SALAD

Grilled chicken breast with mixed greens, cucumbers, green onions, red and yellow peppers, green beans, mango, and wontons with Macadamia nuts and sesame seeds. Tossed in vinaigrette.

NOTE: The mango and the vinaigrette must be removed from this salad. You need to make sure the wontons, which are made from wheat, will combine with the starch in the main entrée.

FACTORY BURRITO GRANDE

Burrito with chicken, cheese, rice, onions, and peppers, topped with guacamole, sour cream, and salsa. Served with black beans and rice.

NOTE: Classic example of too many starches (Group B) in one meal; wheat tortilla, rice, and beans, which is not good. We can only eat one. (Also, avocado is OK but guacamole usually has lemon juice which is not OK. Sour cream and salsa are to be avoided.) There is a lot to take out!

ORANGE CHICKEN

Deep fried chicken breast in a sweet and spicy orange sauce. Served over white rice and garnished with vegetables.

NOTE: Deep fried is tolerable, so here is the problem – "sweet and spicy orange sauce." Also, keep in mind that if you decide to choose the rice, you should pass on the complimentary wheat bread.

CRUSTED CHICKEN ROMANO

Breast of chicken coated with a Romano and Parmesan cheese crust. Served with pasta in tomato sauce.

NOTE: Although tomatoes are acidic, if cooked, tomato sauce is OK. As an alternative, you may ask for olive oil and garlic on your pasta. You may have the complimentary bread and butter since the bread and pasta are made from the same starch – wheat. You can have a salad (no salad dressing; olive oil and salt instead) and/or crab cakes as an appetizer, but stay away from the spicy sauce that comes with it.

REMEMBER: Drink water, sparkling water, or tea without lemon or sugar. And no dessert!

CHICKEN MADEIRA

Sautéed chicken breast topped with asparagus and melted mozzarella cheese, with mushroom Madeira sauce. Served with mashed potatoes.

NOTE: *If you want to have bread and butter or avocado egg rolls as an appetizer, you must substitute the mashed potatoes for spaghetti with garlic and olive oil, since potatoes do not combine with bread or the egg rolls' flour wrapper, which are made from wheat. You may have a salad but remember to stay away from the dressing, pepper, etc., and use olive oil and salt only.*

SHRIMP SCAMPI

Sautéed with garlic, white wine, olive oil, basil, parsley, and tomato. Served with angel hair pasta.

NOTE: *Be sure to ask for no lemon or pepper. You may have the bread and butter that they will put on your table, since bread and pasta are made from the same starch – wheat. You may have a salad and/or avocado egg rolls since they are wrapped in wheat flour tortillas.*

MISO SALMON

With vegetables and steamed rice.

NOTE: *No bread or avocado egg rolls, since they are made with wheat and do not combine with rice. If you want to have the warm bread and butter that they will bring to the table or if you're thinking about ordering the avocado egg rolls, you should have pasta instead of rice, or ask for the salmon on a bed of spinach (without rice). Either way, you may have a salad. No dressing though, olive oil and salt only.*

FILET MIGNON

Served with French fries and onion strings.

NOTE: *French fries are made from potatoes, so, do not combine with the complimentary bread, the avocado egg rolls, or the salad's croutons, since they are all made out of wheat. If you want to have those, you should ask for pasta which is also made out of wheat, instead of the fries.*

REMEMBER: *Drink water, sparkling water, or tea without lemon or sugar. And no dessert!*

GRILLED CHICKEN AND AVOCADO CLUB
Grilled chicken breast with avocado, bacon, tomato, melted Swiss cheese, and herb mayonnaise. Served with French fries.
NOTE: In this sandwich, request no bacon, tomato, or mayonnaise. Also, leave out the French fries (potatoes), since they don't combine with the bread (wheat).

CHICKEN, MUSHROOM, AND ROASTED GARLIC PIZZA
With grilled onions, mozzarella, and Parmesan.
NOTE: You may have the bread and butter, since the bread and pizza are made from the same starch – wheat. You may also have a salad. No dressing though, olive oil and salt only.

ROASTED VEGETABLES AND GOAT CHEESE PIZZA
With roasted Japanese eggplant, red and yellow peppers, grilled onion, artichokes, olives, tomato, and mozzarella.
NOTE: You may have the bread and butter, since the bread and the pasta are made from the same starch – wheat. You may have a salad and/or crab cakes (no sauce) and/or avocado egg rolls since they are wrapped in wheat flour tortillas.

CALIFORNIA PIZZA KITCHEN

PIZZA MARGHERITA
Italian tomatoes and fresh mozzarella cheeses with fresh basil and Parmesan cheese.
NOTE: Tomatoes are acidic, but if they are cooked, it's OK to leave them in. I often ask to add an avocado. A green salad is always a good idea and you know the deal, no dressing; olive oil and salt only.

REMEMBER: *Drink water, sparkling water, or tea without lemon or sugar. And no dessert!*

ROASTED GARLIC CHICKEN PIZZA

Garlic, grilled chicken, mozzarella cheese, onions, and parsley with white wine and garlic-shallot butter.

NOTE: *Although chicken is included in Group A and would combine, I usually substitute it with avocado. Sometimes I have an artichoke dip with pita bread or maybe even a side order of broccoli.*

GRILLED VEGETARIAN SANDWICH

Mushrooms, grilled red and yellow peppers with melted fontina and mozzarella cheeses, baby field greens, sliced Roma tomatoes, and sun-dried tomato aioli. Served with bread: herb-onion focaccia or garlic-cheese focaccia.

NOTE: *If you want to ask for a salad, get it without dressing. Use olive oil and salt only.*

APPLEBEE'S

MOZZARELLA STICKS

Fried and served with marinara sauce.

NOTE: *Tomatoes are acidic, but because they are cooked, it's OK to eat them.*

DYNAMITE SHRIMP

Shrimp coated in bread crumbs and fried, then tossed in a spicy sauce.

NOTE: *Request "sauce on the side" so that you don't have to eat it. Also, since it's prepared with bread crumbs (wheat), you need to make sure it combines with the starch in the main entrée.*

REMEMBER: *Drink water, sparkling water, or tea without lemon or sugar. And no dessert!*

GRILLED CHICKEN CAESAR SALAD

Chicken breast atop a bed of romaine lettuce tossed in garlic Caesar dressing. Topped with challah croutons and shaved Parmesan cheese.

NOTE: Ask for the Caesar dressing on the side and use a minimum amount until you can wean yourself away from it and start using only olive oil and salt. Again, remember that if you want to eat croutons (wheat) you need to make sure it combines with the starch in the main entrée.

BOURBON STREET STEAK

Steak with Cajun spices and served with sautéed onions and mushrooms.

NOTE: Ask for no Cajun spices. It will pay off in the long run. It's much healthier to eat natural foods with no spices at all.

STEAK AND PORTOBELLO

Grilled sirloin steak with sliced, sautéed Portobello mushrooms and brown sauce paired with steamed herb potatoes and seasonal vegetables.

NOTE: Remember to pass on the savory brown sauce! Also, potatoes do not combine with the salad's croutons, or the wheat bread that may be brought to your table, or any other Group B foods.

FRIED CHICKEN

Chicken breast, lightly breaded in seasonings. Served with garlic mashed potatoes, gravy, and seasonal vegetables.

NOTE: The breaded (wheat) chicken does not combine with mashed potatoes. You shouldn't eat the gravy, either. You should cancel the potatoes and ask for pasta which is made out of wheat.

REMEMBER: Drink water, sparkling water, or tea without lemon or sugar. And no dessert!

FISH AND CHIPS

Whitefish fillets, dipped in a light batter and fried; served with fries, cole slaw, and tartar sauce.

NOTE: Forget about cole slaw and tartar sauce; pretend they are not even there. We've got to learn to enjoy the "natural" taste of all foods.

CHICKEN BROCCOLI PASTA ALFREDO BOWL

Grilled or blackened chicken on fettuccine tossed with broccoli and creamy Alfredo sauce. Topped with Parmesan and served with toasted bread.

NOTE: Ask for olive oil (and garlic if you like it!) instead of the Alfredo sauce which is prepared with milk and cream, thus not a good combination. Cream does not combine with meat.

GRILLED SHRIMP PESTO ALFREDO FETTUCCINE

Shrimp tossed with spices and served with basil pesto Alfredo, fettuccine, grape tomatoes, and Italian cheeses; with shaved Parmesan and toasted bread.

NOTE: Tell them to "keep it real" and avoid any spices or tomatoes. It's best to avoid all spices.

BREWTUS STEAK BURGER™

Ten ounces of chopped sirloin burger, topped with cheddar cheese and smoked bacon, and served on a toasted bun.

NOTE: Insist on "no smoked bacon." Never eat pork!

Most of the burgers and sandwiches include fries.

NOTE: Just because they include French fries doesn't mean you must eat them with your sandwich. Having the fries (potato) with bread (wheat) is a Group B combination conflict that should be avoided.

REMEMBER: Drink water, sparkling water, or tea without lemon or sugar. And no dessert!

SUBWAY

Tuna or turkey, cheese, lettuce, olives, avocado, and onions on bread.
NOTE: *Never add sauces, mayonnaise, pepper, vinegar, ketchup, pickles, and of course, never eat pork.*

MCDONALD'S

Cheeseburger, Fillet-O-Fish, or chicken breast sandwich.
NOTE: *Don't eat fries if you want to eat bread. The idea is to choose between wheat or potatoes. If you do want to have French fries (potatoes), you may have the hamburger patty, the fish fillet, or the chicken breast and the other ingredients (lettuce, onions, and melted cheese) but no wheat bun. Be sure to request no pickles or sauce/dressing. It's better to have two hamburgers than one hamburger with French fries.*

Side Salad
Salad Mix: Iceberg lettuce, romaine lettuce, spring mix (may contain baby red romaine, baby green romaine, baby red leaf, baby green leaf, baby red Swiss chard, baby red oak, baby green oak, lolla rossa, tango, tatsoi, arugula, mizuna, radicchio, frisee), carrots, and grape tomatoes.
NOTE: *Be sure to insist on no dressing or seasonings. Also, take out the tomatoes, as they are acidic. Chicken is optional but bacon isn't, so stay away from it. Remember, never eat pork!*

REMEMBER: *Drink water, sparkling water, or tea without lemon or sugar. And no dessert!*

Improvise Anywhere

The Diet is flexible enough that, even if you are at a 7-Eleven in the middle of nowhere, you can still improvise. Here are some suggestions: First - look for any fresh fruit and use it as the base of your meal, taking into consideration the proper combinations; Second - if there are no fresh fruits, try a salad (no dressing) and nuts (without raisins); Third - a bag of nuts (without raisins) and water; crackers are optional and finally – a tuna or turkey sandwich and water.

Points to Remember:
- You can still follow the Gracie Diet when you're eating out.
- Although the food quality may be inferior, you can minimize the harm of restaurant food by modifying your selection to comply with the Gracie Diet food combinations.
- Only eat the bread in the basket if you know that the starch in your main course will be the same as that in the bread.

The Gracie Diet In A Nutshell

- Do not repeat the same food within 24 hrs.
- As you reach and maintain better health, you'll influence everyone around you.
- If you are still hungry after a cooked meal, have seconds. Never eat dessert.

CHAPTER 9:

"Most diseases start in your gut, therefore, fasting is the best medicine."

- Unknown

Detox the Gracie Way

Now that you know how to combine the foods correctly, it's time to learn another important aspect of this program that will give you the elements to complete the cycle of good health: detoxification, or "detox."

Fasting

Uncle Carlos believed that fasting for 24 hours once every month was a good practice, especially for people over the age of forty, since it allowed the body to renew itself through a process known as autophagy, where the cell components, especially the old and damaged ones, were converted into nutrients and be recycled to prolong the survival of the body.

For many years, I have fasted once a month. I choose a day when I know the physical workload will be light, usually on a weekend or in conjunction with travel. I prefer to begin fasting after the second meal of the day because it's usually my heaviest meal and includes cooked foods. I usually have a sensation of hunger about five hours later. So I make a conscious note that it is my body expecting the food it is accustomed to, and I tell myself, "not tonight" and forget it! All I have to do is skip dinner, go to sleep, and in the next morning skip breakfast, and eat again at lunch time. It's important to break your fast with fruits, the purest kind of food. After 24 hours without eating or drinking, you've lost body fluids, so a juicy fruit like watermelon is a great way to replenish yourself. I will get nice big piece, scoop it out with a spoon, suck the juice and spit out the pulp. This process not only allows for better salivation, but also allows you to consume more of the nutrients of the fruit.

Dieting is hard; fasting is even harder. But, the results are worth the effort. The first time you fast the enemy within will use every technique in his arsenal to dissuade you. Remember, he has grown accustomed to mixes of foods that may taste good and satisfy your cravings, but ultimately undermine your health and well-being. So, it's normal to feel a strong reaction to your attempts to change your eating habits and flush your digestive system. You're especially vulnerable to making poor food choices when you're hungry, so be ready for the enemy's best moves – hunger pangs and cravings. If you just can't beat it, then compromise by drinking a glass of water. Over time, you will grow accustomed to the initial discomfort associated with fasting and learn that it quickly passes, especially if you focus on something other than eating.

It is worth noting that the 2016 Nobel Prize of Physiology or Medicine, was awarded to Dr. Yoshinori Ohsumi a researcher from the Tokyo Technology Institute, for his discoveries on the mechanics of autophagy, a fundamental process for degrading and recycling cellular components. The word autophagy originates from the Greek words auto-, meaning "self," and phagein, meaning "to eat." Therefore, autophagy means "self-eating."[6] A 2009 University of Wisconsin study by Professor Richard Weindruch revealed that rhesus monkeys (chosen for their similarity to humans) with reduced calorie diets were significantly healthier with fewer

---

[6]https://www.nobelprize.org/nobel_prizes/medicine/laureates/2016/press.html

cases of diabetes, heart and brain disease, and cancer, and thereby lived a longer, more vital life. Fasting is a great habit to develop. It does wonders for your health – and for your mind.

I urge you to try fasting. Gandhi fasted for weeks at a time, millions do it every day all over the world – some by choice and others out of necessity, and I do it every month. Just do it. You will feel a couple of inches taller, a couple of pounds lighter, and worth an extra million bucks! The benefits of detox through regular fasting will ensure many years of good health, not to mention improving your spirit. You should not fast if you are pregnant, breastfeeding, or taking medicine. When you detach from eating simply as a habit you discover a surprising truth: Sometimes the best meal is the one you don't eat!

The Lime Regimen
I once asked Uncle Carlos how he determined the proper food combinations. He related two contradicting stories about the value of limes. One expert convincingly argued that the lime was bad for your health. Yet, another expert presented an equally convincing argument lauding the benefits of eating limes. Who was right? Carlos concluded, "They were both correct – the secret was in how to consume the lime." Lime is highly alkaline when you consume it by itself as a standalone meal. However, if combined with any other food – salad, fish, drinks – it becomes highly acidic and very detrimental to your health! To tap the healing power of this fruit, Carlos developed the lime regimen to cleanse and alkalinize the body.

Warning: Use the Lime Regimen only after following the diet for at least six months and ensure you adhere to the diet's recommended food combinations (see the Gracie Diet Table of Combinations on pages 80-82).

The Cleansing Program

Take the following doses of plain lime juice as the first complete meal of the day. Ensure you have enough limes on hand to complete the regimen without interruption.

1- With your hand, press the limes on the counter to soften them.
2- Wash, cut, juice, and strain the fruit using non-metallic utensils.
3- Use a measuring cup to ensure accurate dosages.
4- Immediately consume the extracted and strained juice.
5- You may add fresh coconut water to make it more palatable. Do not use commercially packaged coconut water.
6- Use a straw to protect your teeth and drink slowly, especially when drinking large amounts of juice.
7- Wait for at least five hours before eating lunch.
8- After lunch, wait at least 4 ½ hours before eating dinner.
9- Refrain from eating other acidic fruit or substance (kefir, yogurt); fried foods; refined sugar; milk or curdled milk; aged cheeses; dried legumes (beans, lentils, chickpeas, etc.).
10- Do not consume alcohol or smoke during the regimen (or ever for that matter).

Frequency: If you have been following the Gracie Diet for at least six months, do this regimen once a year.

Dosage Guidelines

Day	Quantity
1	50 ml
2	100 ml
3	150 ml
4	150 ml
5	200 ml
6	200 ml
7	250 ml
8	300 ml
9	300 ml
10	350 ml
11	350 ml
12	300 ml
13	300 ml
14	250 ml
15	200 ml
16	200 ml
17	150 ml
18	150 ml
19	100 ml
20	50 ml

Note: If you are not ready, or choose not to do the full 20-day regimen, you could prepare a breakfast meal of 150 ml of lime juice (adding fresh coconut water is optional) two or three times a month. Then, wait five hours before eating lunch. This is a great way to strengthen your immune system.

Obstipation

The symptoms of obstipation, or chronic constipation, are: defecating less than three times a week; hard feces in small volume and difficult or painful defecation; a sensation of incomplete evacuation; and frequent use of laxatives, suppositories, and enemas. It can cause abdominal swelling and pain, irritability, flatulence, and hemorrhoids. It may contribute to the development of appendicitis, colon cancer, obesity, and diabetes. According to the American College of Gastroenterology, obstipation is one of the Western world's most common gastrointestinal maladies. It is the most common digestive problem in the USA, responsible for 2.5 million office visits, 92,000 hospitalizations, and the purchase of hundreds of millions of dollars in laxatives. An average of 900 people die every year from diseases associated with constipation, with women suffering from the condition at a ratio three times higher than men.

The Digestive Process

Food passes through the mouth, down the esophagus into the stomach. The stomach liquefies the food and passes it to the small intestine, a long, sinuous tube through which the body absorbs nutrients. The body uses these nutrients to fuel all of its functions. Unused food becomes feces, and moves to the large intestine or colon as a liquid. The large intestine extracts water from the liquid feces transforming it into solid waste as it moves toward the rectum. When the feces reaches the end of the rectum, it places pressure on the anal sphincter muscle. This pressure tells the brain that it's time to defecate. If the brain agrees, then the sphincter relaxes and the body eliminates the feces.

Problems arise when the brain tells the sphincter to "hold it for later." The body continues to extract water from the feces while it remains inside the rectum causing it to harden. As the body digests more food, feces accumulates in the rectum. The longer the body holds the feces, the more it accumulates and hardens leading to discomfort and potentially serious consequences. When the brain eventually allows defecation, passing the hardened fecal mass could be painful. Using laxatives or other unnatural forms of intestinal regulation is a poor solution as it can cause dependency, unnecessarily exposes your body to more chemicals, and is expensive. There is a better way.

Drink a glass of water when you awaken. We eliminate water during sleep through breathing, sweating, urination, and absorption. A glass of water first thing in the morning primes the system and facilitates the evacuation process. Drinking water throughout the day between meals also helps.

Eat healthily. Follow the Gracie Diet Table of Combinations (pages 80-82). If constipated, choose oats; Malabar spinach; squash; fennel; chicory; oily fruits like avocado, olives, fresh coconuts (water and flesh); and fruits like prunes, figs, papayas, oranges, tangerines, grapes, watermelon, and pears. Start with the 14-day meal plan (pages 132-135). Try fruit meals for breakfast and dinner, and a cooked meal at lunch when your metabolism is most active.

Establish a routine. The ideal routine is to completely evacuate once daily in the morning after breakfast. But, if your brain tells you it's time to go, then find a bathroom – never "hold it for later." The more you "hold it," the more you confuse the messages from your excretory system. To establish the morning routine, sit on the toilet after breakfast until you receive the message. In the beginning, this may take ten to fifteen minutes. Massage your tummy in a circular motion while you wait. If you can't defecate within fifteen minutes, don't worry about it. But, maintain the daily routine until your body forms the habit.

Posture. Scientists at the Stanford University Pelvic Floor Clinic explain that the human body is designed to evacuate from a crouched position. This position removes pressure from the rectum, allowing more natural and efficient evacuation. If you've ever defecated outdoors, then you are probably familiar with this position. In fact, toilets in many parts of the world are designed for this position. When using a chair-style toilet, try to elevate your knees to achieve a crouch-like position.

Be physically active. Regularly participate in some kind of physical activity such as walking, bike riding, or dancing to promote regularity.

Diarrhea

The symptoms of diarrhea are soft or watery stool and frequent need to defecate. Follow the Gracie Diet Table of Combinations (pages 80-82) with foods that your intestines will retain longer, such as rice, potatoes, yams, guava, sweet apples, bananas, pomegranate, chestnuts, peppermint tea, and black tea. Avoid sweets and fat.

Science Alert cited a study on Parkinson's disease published in *Cell* suggesting the disease might start in the gut, not the brain. This may explain reports of constipation and other digestive problems up to ten years prior to the onset of tremors.

"We have discovered for the first time a biological link between the gut microbiome and Parkinson's disease," said lead researcher Sarkis Mazmanian from the California Institute of Technology (Caltech).

"More generally, this research reveals that a neurodegenerative disease may have its origins in the gut, and not only in the brain as had been previously thought." [7]

> **Eating Every Other Day**
> Mark Mattson, a researcher at the National Institute on Aging in Baltimore, Maryland, thinks an alternate route may be through what he calls intermittent fasting. Health benefits in mice that eat only every other day are similar to those for mice that eat a calorie-restricted diet—they live 30 percent longer, Mattson says. And, he adds, "We see vast improvements in variables that indicate risk of disease." Mattson's objective is not weight loss (though the ad hoc fasters happily report pounds lost, as well as other health benefits including reduced allergy sensitivity and more energy). Nor is Mattson especially interested in extending life span. Instead, he wants to boost what he calls the human "health span"—the period of a life in which a person enjoys good health, even into their eighties or nineties.

Points to Remember:
- After 40 years of age, practice fasting once a month. It's better to break the fast with a fruit meal.
- Do the Lime Regimen once a year.
- Develop the habit of going to the bathroom in the morning after breakfast. Never "hold for later" the need to evacuate.

---

[7] http://www.sciencealert.com/new-evidence-suggests-parkinsons-might-start-in-the-gut-before-spreading-to-the-brain

The Gracie Diet In A Nutshell

- Chew your meal well to facilitate the action of the enzymes over the foods, and the assimilation of the nutrients.
- At meal time, focus on the food. Avoid reading, talking on the phone, or watching television.
- Whenever possible, take a 15- to 30-minute nap after lunch.

CHAPTER 10:

"One should eat to live, not live to eat."
— Moliere

Tips for Losing Weight

To optimize digestion, increase energy, and have a long healthy life, you must space your meals appropriately and properly combine your foods at each sitting. However, if weight loss is your primary goal, you will need to go one step further. You will need to control your caloric intake and minimize the consumption of certain foods, and in order to do that you will need to develop a very high level of self-control.

How to Acquire the Gracie "Iron Will"

The Gracie Diet is a great opportunity to develop the priceless habit of self-discipline. I learned from my father at an early age that every meal was a chance to practice self-control. Sometimes it was a question of me having three slices of toast instead of four. Or two scoops of ice cream instead of three. Why not one more slice of toast or another scoop of ice cream? Because you're no longer hungry! When I felt like overeating, more often than not I was being led by the anticipation of how good the food would taste. In other words, pleasure was the driving force behind that extra slice or the extra scoop. There came a time when I could tell myself: "Okay, I will have another slice and one more scoop – but not today!" That was a major revelation. Confronting the temptation and then denying it caused the craving to vanish. It made me stronger. It put me in control. It increased my self-worth. Not only is this self-mastery the single most important element of the weight-loss equation, but it will positively impact every aspect of your life.

Calorie Control

Calories are measurements of energy: 3,500 calories equals one pound of fat. So, burning 3,500 calories means losing one pound of fat. When it comes to weight loss, there is one more equation that matters: You must burn more calories than you consume. Men between the ages of 19-50 should consume between 2,200 and 2,600 calories per day. Women 19-50 should consume between 1,800 and 2,200 per day. The more active you are, the higher your metabolism will be, and the more calories you will burn.

John O. Holloszy of the Washington University School of Medicine, in St. Louis, Missouri, and his colleagues cataloged what they call "profound and sustained beneficial effects" of the calorie-restricted diet. The dietitian-approved meal plan was enlivened by a nutrient-dense array of fruits, vegetables, legumes, and whole grains (*Proceedings of the National Academy of Sciences*). Holloszy says:

> The calorie-restriction subjects scored vastly better on all major risk factors for heart disease including total cholesterol, triglycerides, and blood pressure. Each of these tends to increase with advancing age. They also have very low amounts of body fat compared to the average person in the control group, who had about 25 percent body fat. This quality protects the calorie restrictors from the type 2 diabetes associated with obesity.[8]

Play This Game at Your Next Meal

As a great way to begin developing your discipline while monitoring your food consumption, do this at your next

---

[8] http://www.pnas.org/content/101/17/6659.long

meal. Find something that you really enjoy eating and tell yourself, "I will only eat three-fourths of it!" If you can "win" this game, you will take a major step forward in developing your personal discipline and healthy eating habits. You'll be amazed at how easily you can trim your meals and achieve great results with less food. A golden rule is to stop eating when you are 80% full. Just remember, you'll be eating again in about 4 ½ hours anyway. Eating less at each meal is good for your body and your mind! I can't overemphasize enough how practicing dietary discipline will enhance your overall health. You simply won't believe how it will improve your ability to achieve your personal goals.

A Surefire Way to Burn Fat
In addition to monitoring your caloric intake, one great way to help you reach your weight-loss goal is to make one-fruit-meals part of your routine. Once a day, have a meal in which you limit yourself to a single fruit. You may have as much of the one fruit as you want, but you must eat only the one fruit – without bread or cheese. Be sure to eat enough to tide you over until the next meal. This may take some practice, since most people aren't accustomed to eating four or five bananas or half a watermelon in one sitting. Since you are only eating one kind of fruit, you may feel hungry before the 4 ½ hours are up. No worries — drink a glass of water and your hunger pangs will subside! Your body will soon grow accustomed to the regimen. Remember: Don't have the same fruit again for 24 hours.

Managing Your Carbohydrates
The extreme popularity of the Atkins, South Beach, and other low-carbohydrate diets led many people to believe that carbohydrates are the primary cause of the obesity

epidemic. That's a dangerous oversimplification, similar to "fat is bad." Don't be misled by these broad pronouncements on the dangers of carbohydrates. They are an extremely important part of a healthy diet. Carbohydrates are the most common source of energy found in food, and they are vital in promoting proper organ function. The key is to understand the difference between complex carbohydrates or "good carbs," and simple carbohydrates, "bad carbs." Easily digestible simple carbohydrates from white bread, white rice, pastries, sugared sodas, and other highly processed foods may, indeed, contribute to weight gain among other negative consequences to your health. On the other hand, complex carbohydrates from whole grains, beans, fruits, and vegetables deliver minerals, fiber, and a host of essential vitamins. If you're trying to lose weight, eliminate all refined grains from your diet, since they are stripped of all their nutrients and break down quickly making the pancreas work hard to churn out insulin for energy – a danger for those at risk of diabetes. Stick to minimally processed whole grains, fruits, and vegetables and you'll be good to go!

Protein Sources
Also known as the building block of life, protein's most important role is to build, maintain, and replace tissue in our bodies. Protein is a long chain of amino acids linked together. Our muscles, organs, and some of our hormones are made up of mostly protein. Our body is able to produce some of the amino acids (protein) we need. The rest (known as essential amino acids) must be obtained through our diets. Since I choose not to eat red meat, people often ask where I get my protein. Some of the best sources of protein are: avocados, beans, nuts, and fish. You may add chicken or red meat, but scientific studies have proven that a diet de-

rived exclusively from vegetables can provide all the essential amino acids for optimal health. This means you can get all the protein you need without the cholesterol and toxins found in animal products.

Fat Facts
Fat is a necessary nutrient and most foods contain some type of fat. Fat helps in our energy production and our blood clotting; it helps regulate blood pressure and to maintain a healthy nervous system; and your skin, hair, and nails all depend on it. But, some fats are better for you than others, so it is critical that you know the difference between healthy, good fats, and unhealthy, bad fats. The good fats include the following: monounsaturated fat (olives, avocados, nuts), polyunsaturated fat (vegetable oils, cereals, bananas, hemp seeds) and omega-3 fatty acids (fish, flax, walnuts). Then there are the bad fats, and they include: saturated fat (animal products such as meat, dairy, and eggs), trans fat (hydrogenated oils found in cookies, crackers, cakes, and also common in fried foods) and cholesterol (animal products, dairy, organs). Although all fats are okay in moderation, if you're trying to lose weight and reach optimum health, it is best to stick to the good fats and minimize the rest.

How to Lose Weight and Still Occasionally Enjoy Alcohol
Our lifestyle prohibits alcohol consumption, so it's not part of the Gracie Diet. However, if drinking is part of your lifestyle, then follow the proper food combining guidelines when choosing your beverage. Your eventual goal should be to wean off alcohol altogether, but until that happens, consider reducing the frequency of your consumption. If you normally drink every weekend, start by cutting it back to every other weekend, and then down to once a month.

Eventually, when you begin to feel the positive results of all the other dietary changes you are making, and your confidence is growing from living a healthier lifestyle, you will find greater satisfaction in resisting the temptation than you do from drinking, and that's when you'll be able to quit completely and feel great about it!

Alcohol consumption is your choice. Many people imbibe for a wide variety of reasons. To each his own. I choose not to drink alcohol. I never saw my parents drinking alcohol, and their personal example has influenced me to avoid the practice to this day. More important, I know that the example I set for my children influences their choices and that my actions speak much louder than words. I believe the consequences of alcohol consumption – near-term and long-term – are unpredictable. I would rather not risk a negative outcome when it comes to my health or that of my children. Choosing the alcohol-free path will be one of the best decisions you'll ever make.

> **How to Stay True to the Gracie Diet**
> What do you do when someone prepares a meal for you that does not comply with the Gracie Diet? How do you handle a big Thanksgiving dinner full of incompatible food combinations or a celebration where everyone is drinking alcohol (and lots of it)? First, make a positive choice. Follow the course of action that will make you feel good about yourself. If you make an exception to the Gracie dietary guidelines, then do it because you feel that it's the right thing to do. Ask yourself which will make you feel better, avoiding unhealthy food selections or pleasing your host? Of course, you should do it tactfully, respectfully, and confidently. Often, it's easiest for

everyone if you just employ a simple excuse – like you're not feeling well or you're allergic to certain foods or beverages. Just be aware that what's at stake here is something much larger than the momentary circumstance. As a child, I never saw my father or other members of my family smoke or drink – and I'm sure they were conscious of the positive influence this would have on me.

Points to Remember:
- The quality of your weight-loss plan doesn't matter if you lack the discipline to follow it.
- If weight loss is your goal, manage your caloric intake and always leave the table knowing that you could eat more.
- If you like carbonation, drink sparkling water. Never drink sodas.

 The Gracie Diet In A Nutshell

- Start your meal by eating the salad first.
- Only use extra virgin olive oil and salt on your salad. Never use lemon sauces or vinegar.
- Drink alcohol if you must, but understand the health and safety risks and remember that eating right is the most important activity in your life.

CHAPTER 11:

"It doesn't matter how many times you fall but how many times you get up."

― Abraham Lincoln

The Role of Exercise

Physical exercise – and especially its relationship to diet – is an important but commonly misunderstood component of a healthy lifestyle. The most common misconception is that you must adopt a rigorous workout routine in order to lose weight. How the body reacts to different types of exercises depends on many factors. The key is to find the right exercise for you. More is not necessarily better. The idea that weight control is linked to exercise is seemingly obvious. In all areas of our lives, we see that work brings results and hard work usually brings even better results. But with regard to weight control, research proves that more is not better.

Dr. Wayne Miller and colleagues at George Washington University Medical Center conducted a survey of 493 weight-loss studies. The purpose was to determine whether the addition of aerobic exercise to a restricted-calorie diet accelerated weight loss. The research showed that diet and moderate aerobic exercise provide only a small improvement in weight loss compared to diet alone.

An Appalachian State University study focused on a group of 91 obese women organized into four groups. The first group followed a restricted diet of 1,200 to 1,300 calories per day; group two had no diet restrictions but performed aerobic exercise for 45 minutes, five days each week; the third group combined exercise and diet. The women in the fourth group acted as controls and followed their normal daily routines. Although they exercised for almost four hours each week, the exercise-only group lost just three pounds. The women combining diet and exercise got the best results, losing a combined 16 pounds of fat. But this was only one pound more than the group on the diet alone. The researchers stated that aerobic exercise had only "minor, insignificant effect" on fat loss.

For exercise to have a real impact on your weight, you would need to follow a strict regimen for a long time. It's always easier said than done. For most of us, strong intentions and high motivation quickly erode in the face of demanding daily workouts. The good news is that it's not a disaster if you ease up on the exercise, as long as you keep doing something. While diet is more effective than exercise in weight management, it's still important to exercise. The real problems arise only when people completely stop exercising. I offer three points to guide you in whatever exercise program you choose to follow: make it fun, start slowly, and keep climbing.

Make It Fun

Find an exercise that interests you. The problem with most aerobic workouts is that they are incredibly boring. Few people can sustain the motivation to ride a stationary bicycle or climb a StairMaster for weeks or months in order to see any benefits. To be sure, some motivate themselves by challenging their bodies and minds to the max in every workout. Elite athletes do this by reaching their physical limit and staying there for as long as possible. If possible, they would probably remain at that point all the time. Monotony is not a problem because they turn every session into a competition. But most of us are not elite athletes with the accompanying obsessive mindset. As a result, it's only a matter of time before we burn out. That's why it's best if exercise is a byproduct of an exciting or enjoyable activity instead of the main focus. For example, our training at the Gracie Jiu-Jitsu Academy doesn't include calisthenics or weight-lifting, but the students are shedding pounds without even realizing it because they are so consumed with learning the techniques. Whether you choose jiu-jitsu, basketball, or just a brisk walk through a pleasant neighborhood, the important thing is that it stimulates you beyond the fitness aspect so that you can sustain the activity for a lifetime.

Start Slowly
Your exercise should be moderately challenging. The key to weight loss is to find the right balance of time and exertion that you can sustain given your personal schedule, interests, and physical abilities. Workout for as long and as hard as you like, but understand that after approximately the first fifteen minutes, there's a sharp drop off in the positive effects of exercise. Exercising for an hour doesn't mean you'll get twice the effect of exercising for thirty minutes. You will surely benefit, but the return on your effort diminishes over time. It's much more important, therefore, to be consistent and comfortable than to "knock yourself out." I recommend brisk walking, especially with a partner, for weight control and overall health. If you take a thirty-minute walk every day at a fast but comfortable pace, that will give you virtually all the benefits that you'd get from a more strenuous (and less pleasant) workout. And if you take the walk with someone whose company you enjoy, the time will pass very quickly.

Keep Climbing
The real goal of exercising today should be to want to do it again tomorrow. No matter how good a workout is one day – or one week, or even for a whole month – you will lose the

benefits unless you continue your exercise over a much longer time period. In fact, your goal should be finding an activity that you can enjoy for the rest of your life. The reason so many people are so passionate about Gracie Jiu-Jitsu is because anyone can do it and you never stop getting better. Even at 95 my father was still experimenting with new techniques! If you already have a regular exercise routine, that's great. If you don't, start with a 20-minute walk three times a week.

Keep a calendar of your exercise schedule and increase one digit on either side of your routine every two weeks. From a 20-minute walk three times a week, go to 30 minutes three times a week, or 20 minutes four times a week. Then break up the routine by expanding to include one new exercise – like sit-ups or push-ups – every two weeks. Gradually increase the number of repetitions, and every two weeks add an entirely new exercise. The quick, positive health benefits of this exercise will have you so motivated that you'll be amazed at how much more you want to do. It's definitely a great feeling – but don't just depend on a short-term high. Remember, you're not training for a sprint; you're training for a long, healthy life. Expect an occasional fall along the way. It happens to everyone. You win every time you pick yourself up and continue forward.

> **How do supplements work with the Diet?**
> We don't endorse supplements. Even those that claim to be natural are produced in a laboratory using potentially harmful chemicals. See an article published by the *World Journal of Hepatology* entitled "Acute liver injury induced by weight-loss herbal supplements." documenting the results of a study by the Gastroenterology and Pathology Department at UCLA Harbor Medical Center.[10] The Gracie Diet will optimize your health so you don't need supplements. A well-balanced diet with a good variety of fruits and vegetables, nuts and grains will provide all the nutrients you need.

Points to Remember:
- In order to be sustainable, exercise can't be "a means to an end." It should be fun and rewarding in its own right.
- Find an exercise program that's reasonably challenging, not overwhelming.
- A simple and convenient initial program is to take 20- to 30-minute walks three times a week. The benefits are incredible!

---

[10] Chen GC, Ramanathan VS, Law D, et al. "Acute liver injury induced by weight-loss herbal supplements." *World Journal of Hepatology.* 2010;2(11):410-415. doi:10.4254/wjh.v2.i11.410.)

The Gracie Diet In A Nutshell

- Cigarettes kill. If you smoke, try to find out why, and quit!
- Do not consume alcohol, sodas, or processed liquids.
- Children will drink what the parents put in the refrigerator.

CHAPTER 12:

"Let food be thy medicine and medicine be thy food."
- *Hippocrates*

Final Considerations
- Raw or cooked egg yolk, coconut water, brewer's yeast, coffee, and several kinds of tea are neutral. They're compatible with any food.
- Bread should be made from whole flour and should not be consumed within 24 hours of being baked. Then, prior to being eaten, it should be toasted or oven-warmed.
- Avoid sweets, canned foods in syrup, and spices including: pepper, clove, cinnamon, mustard, pickles, and vinegar.
- Don't eat pork in any form.
- Space meals at least 4½ hours apart to ensure complete digestion before you eat again. It's OK to wait longer. Young children may eat every 4 hours. If you feel hungry before it's time to eat, drink water or fresh coconut water. Never snack!
- The digestive process starts in the mouth, therefore, chewing your food well is extremely important, just like salivating the fruit juices before ingesting them.

Group A: Meats, Seafood, Legumes, Vegetables, and Cooked Foods
- It's best to eat cooked food at home where you can monitor food quality, ensure proper preparation, and guarantee proper hygiene.
- The problem with restaurant food is the heavy use of condiments, spices, and sauces, which changes the real taste of the foods and could adversely affect food combinations

and meal digestibility.
- When eating out, order the food as plain as possible, always requesting the dressing or sauces on the side so that you can use it less and less, or not at all. It's always better to only use extra virgin olive oil and salt.
- Eat as many fresh and colorful vegetables and dark leafy greens as possible.
- Avoid drinking too much water with your meal. It's better to drink it before the meal.
- Try to eat your cooked meal in the afternoon when your metabolism is more active, thereby making it easier to digest.
- The strongest animals, and those with most endurance, do not eat meat.
- Groups C, D, E, and F do not combine with Group A.
- When cheese is melted, it falls under Group A.
- When the banana is baked or cooked, it can be eaten with either Group A or Group C.
- Avoid aluminum pans and utensils.

Group B: Starches Do Not Combine With Each Other
- Eat only one starch per meal. For example: Do not eat rice with beans. Beans do not combine with corn or wheat tortillas; French fries (potatoes) do not combine with a sandwich (wheat); yet pasta combines with bread, pizza and/or lasagna, because they are all derived from the same starch – wheat.
- Starches, if not prepared with fat (butter/oil), can be combined with sweet fruits and fresh cheeses (Group C) i.e. toast (wheat) with fresh cheese, watermelon juice and dates or honey.
- If you want to lose weight, cut down on your starch consumption, especially refined grains.
- Read the ingredients when you choose breads. Some mix

several grains, or are loaded with oils and fats. Rye crackers are a great alternative to white bread!

Group C: Sweet Fruits and Foods, and Fresh Cheeses.
- All sweet fruits combine with each other and one food from Group B (Starches), if not prepared with fat, such as butter.
- Use dates, honey, and raisins as a way to satisfy your sweet tooth.
- Dried sweet fruits also combine with fresh sweet fruits, i.e. dried pears/papaya/grapes, etc.
- When mixing sweet fruits (Group C) with raw bananas (Group E) remember to not eat starches (Group B), because they don't combine with bananas.
- Have fun experimenting with various sweet fruit combinations for juice blends and smoothies.
- You can juice the fruits or eat them in their natural state. In many cases, if you extract and consume only the vitamin-rich juice you will increase the nutritional value of the meal.
- Choose the white fresh cheeses, cream, ricotta, cottage, etc. Avoid aged cheeses like Roquefort, Camembert, etc., as well as spicy cheeses.
- A healthier alternative to cheeses in general, especially with a Group C meal, is the meat of fresh coconut.

Group D: Acidic Foods
- Never mix one kind of acidic fruit with any another food, including other acidic fruits.
- Eat enough at one sitting to hold you over until the next meal.
- Do not eat acidic fruits that have been dried, i.e. peaches, pineapples, apricots, oranges, berries, etc., since they are often sweetened in the process. However, if they are naturally dried with no sweetener of any kind, they may be

eaten by themselves.
- It's always better to eat acidic fruits for breakfast, since that will ensure complete digestion of your last meal.
- It's best not to eat acidic fruits more than two times a week.
- Lime must be treated as a remedy, and should only be consumed by itself. The only exception is adding fresh coconut water to make it more palatable.

Group E: Bananas for Sure!
- Extremely nutritious, easy to find, and full of healthy benefits.
- Raw bananas combine with all fresh sweet fruits and fresh cheeses (Group C).
- When having bananas in a Group C meal, do not include starches (Group B).
- They combine with milk (Group F).
- A meal of only bananas (or any other single fruit) will help you lose weight.
- Cooked or baked bananas combine with Groups A, B, C.

Group F: Milk
- Milk is beneficial only for children during their growing years.
- Once you reach adulthood, the less milk you drink, the better.
- Milk combines with bread (Group B), butter, and cheese; with cereal (some cereals should be avoided because of their ingredients); or bananas (Group E).
- Do not drink milk with meats or vegetables (Group A) or with fruits (Groups C and D).

The Gracie Diet 14-Day Meal Plan
I realize that most of these meals will be completely new to you and may seem unfamiliar, unappetizing, or even intimidating. I urge you to try each of them before you pass judgment on the Diet. View the experience as a visit to a new

place or learning a new language. Approach the Diet with curiosity and an open mind. It will take a bit of practice, but the benefits are worth it. The habit of eating with a wholesome purpose will put you, your children, and your loved ones on a new path toward health and happiness.

The following 14-day plan is a good place to start. It contains recipes that the Gracie family has used for many years. They're delicious and easy to prepare. I have prepared all of them by myself many times. If I can do it, so can you! At our house we usually eat at least one sweet meal (Group C), often two, each day. We've arranged our lives so that we eat our primary cooked meal (Group A) for lunch. Since the body's metabolism is more active during the day, this makes the cooked meal easier to digest. I realize that for many families having the primary cooked meal during the day is unfeasible due to school, work, and other scheduling conflicts. It's no problem having the main meal (Group A) at night. It's still a good idea to try some fruit meals (Group C and B optional) for dinner, and assess how you and your family like it, not to mention that the clean-up is much quicker!

Following are samples of meals that adhere to the Gracie Diet combination guidelines. As you experiment with these meals, you can substitute one food for another of the same group, or you can add another food to the meal so long as it doesn't violate a combination principle for that particular group. Some meals will be familiar to you and some will be completely new. Although eating a variety of foods is best, if you find a set of breakfasts, lunches, and dinners that you take a particular liking to, you can repeat them as often as you'd like. Just don't eat the same food within 24 hours.

Experiment with these meals, develop new tastes, appreciate the variety and flexibility, but most of all understand that they will improve your health. Imagine that you are a VIP guest on some exotic island for a two-week vacation and this is what your hosts served you each day. Rejoice!

GRACIE DIET

	BREAKFAST	LUNCH
MON	Oatmeal (**B**) and raisins, dates or honey (**C**) and apple juice (**C**).	**Salad:** Lettuce, broccoli, avocado, radish, onions, beats, cucumber, celery, bell peppers, hearts of palm, sprout, arugula, etc.(**A**). Olive oil and salt only. Add cashews, walnuts, Brazil nuts, Macadamia, etc.(**A**).
TUE	Bananas (**E**) blended with cantaloupe juice (**C**); a teaspoon of cream cheese (**C**) is optional.	**Salad:** Same as above.
WED	Eggs (**A**), whole grain toast (**B**), and butter (**A**) with coffee/tea (neutral); no sugar or lemon, artificial sweetener OK.	**Salad:** Same as above.
THUR	Mangos (**D**); peel, suck the juice, and spit out the pulp.	**Salad:** Same as above.
FRI	Bananas (**E**) blended with watermelon juice (**C**).	**Salad:** Same as above.
SAT	Vegetable Juice (see page 173) with avocado (**A**) on toasted sourdough/whole grain bread (**B**).	**Salad:** Same as above.
SUN	Oranges (**D**) juiced; or peel them, suck the juice, and spit out the pulp.	**Salad:** Same as above.

14-DAY MEAL PLAN

WEEK 1

LUNCH	DINNER
Entrée: Baked salmon with rosemary (**A**), quinoa (**B**), and cream of spinach - use quinoa flour (**A-B**). **Drink:** Regular or sparkling water (no lemon), coconut water (neutral), or carrot juice (**A**); adding some of the salad ingredients (**A**) to the juice is optional.	Watermelon juice (**C**), cottage cheese (**C**), rye bread (**B**); raisins, dates, or honey (**C**) are optional.
Entrée: Chicken stroganoff (**A**), brown rice (**B**), and onion quiche - use rice flour (**A-B**). **Drink:** Same as above.	Vegetable Juice (see page 173) with avocado (**A**) on toasted sourdough/whole grain bread (**B**).
Entrée: Fish soufflé (**A**), whole wheat pasta (**B**), and steamed/cooked vegetables (**A**). **Drink:** Same as above.	Apple juice (**C**), cottage cheese (**C**), and rye crackers (**B**); raisins, dates or honey (**C**) are optional.
Entrée: Corn soup (**A**) and grilled Monterey Jack cheese (**A**) on sourdough/whole grain bread (**B**). **Drink:** Same as above.	Honeydew melon juice (**C**), fresh coconut meat (**C**), and whole grain crackers (**B**).
Entrée: Baked fish a la coconut (**A**), brown rice (**B**), and eggplant quiche - use rice flour (**A-B**). **Drink:** Same as above.	Sweet pears (**C**); raisins, dates, or honey (**C**) are optional.
Entrée: Round roast (**A**), whole wheat pasta (**B**), and cream of corn - use wheat flour (**A-B**). **Drink:** Same as above.	Cantaloupe pieces (**C**), sweet grapes (**C**), and bananas (**E**).
Entrée: Shrimp (**A**) and potato (**B**) combo, potato chips/ French fries (**B**), and steamed/sautéed vegetables (**A**). **Drink:** Same as above.	Fresh figs (**C**), ricotta (**C**), and honey (**C**).

GRACIE DIET

	BREAKFAST	LUNCH
MON	Milk (**F**) and grilled Monterey Jack cheese (**A**) on sourdough/ whole grain bread (**B**).	**Salad:** Lettuce, broccoli, avocado, radish, onions, beats, cucumber, celery, bell peppers, hearts of palm, sprout, arugula, etc.(**A**). Olive oil and salt only. Add cashews, walnuts, Brazil nuts, Macadamia, etc.(**A**).
TUE	Bananas (**E**) blended with honeydew melon juice (**C**).	**Salad:** Same as above.
WED	Papaya (**C**), cream cheese (**C**); raisins, dates, or honey (**C**) are optional.	**Salad:** Same as above.
THUR	Sweet pears (**C**), cantaloupe (**C**), dates, or honey (**C**) are optional.	**Salad:** Same as above.
FRI	Bananas (**E**) blended with apple juice (**C**).	**Salad:** Same as above.
SAT	Tangerines (**D**); peel them, suck the juice, and spit out the pulp.	**Salad:** Same as above.
SUN	Milk (**F**) blended with bananas (**E**).	**Salad:** Same as above.

14-DAY MEAL PLAN

WEEK 2

LUNCH	DINNER
Entrée: Grilled chicken (**A**), quinoa (**B**), and zucchini quiche - use quinoa flour (**A-B**). **Drink:** Regular or sparkling water (no lemon), coconut water (neutral), or carrot juice (**A**); adding some of the salad ingredients (**A**) to the juice is optional.	Red apples (**C**), papaya (**C**), cottage cheese (**C**), and bananas (**E**).
Entrée: Grilled halibut (**A**), baked potatoes (**B**), and steamed/sautéed vegetables (**A**). **Drink:** Same as above	Persimmons (**C**) and cottage cheese (**C**); rye crackers (**B**) are optional.
Entrée: Squash soup (**A**) and grilled Monterey Jack cheese (**A**) sandwich on sourdough/whole grain bread (**B**). **Drink:** Same as above	Sweet grape juice (**C**), fresh coconut meat (**C**), and whole grain toast (**B**).
Entrée: Fish soufflé (**A**), brown rice (**B**), and sautéed green beans (**A**). **Drink:** Same as above	Vegetable Juice (see page 173) with avocado (**A**) on toasted sourdough/whole grain bread (**B**).
Entrée: Onion quiche - use wheat flour (**A-B**), whole wheat pasta (**B**), and cream of spinach - use wheat flour (**A-B**). **Drink:** Same as above	Watermelon juice (**C**), Monterey Jack cheese – not melted (**C**), and whole grain crackers (**B**).
Entrée: Baked fish a la coconut (**A**), brown rice (**B**), and steamed/sautéed vegetables (**A**). **Drink:** Same as above	Cantaloupe juice (**C**), blended with pure açaí (**C**), and honey or dates (**C**).
Entrée: Steak (**A**), mashed potatoes (**B**), and corn on the cob (**A**). **Drink:** Same as above	Honeydew melon juice (**C**), cream cheese (**C**), and whole grain crackers (**B**).

> **The Secret**
>
> Efficiency in combat is what has put my family on the map, efficiency in health and nutrition is what made it possible. The healthy lifestyle taught to me by my uncle and father is the greatest gift I ever received, and it is, without a doubt, the greatest gift I have ever given my children. I am happy to finally share with you the only self-defense system greater than Gracie Jiu-Jitsu, the Gracie Diet. Like any street fight, the fight for optimum health will not be an easy one. Things will not always go according to plan, and undoubtedly, you will get hit. As long as you can remain focused, stay strong, and stick to the plan, victory is yours!

Points to Remember:
- Foods prepared with fat, oil, or butter, (Group A) do not combine with sugar, sweets, or fruits (Group C).
- If you have a sweet tooth, satisfy your craving with a Group C meal.
- If you want to lose weight, try meals of only one kind of fruit. Start once a week and gradually increase until you get to three or four meals a week. Be sure to vary your fruits.

The Gracie Diet In A Nutshell

- Drink a glass of water every day as soon as you wake up.
- Sunbathe at a healthy time and wear sunscreen.
- Flexibility will keep you young. Stretch every day.

ENTRÉES MENU INDEX

1	Onion Quiche
2	Zucchini Quiche
3	Eggplant Quiche
4	Chicken Stroganoff
5	Chicken Soup
6	Cream of Spinach
7	Cream of Corn
8	Chayote Squash Soufflé
9	Fish Soufflé
10	Baked Fish a la Coconut
11	Baked Salmon with Rosemary
12	Fresh Codfish and Potato Casserole
13	Shrimp Hungarian Style
14	Shrimp and Potato Combo
15	Shrimp Linguine
16	Gluten-Free Quiche
17	Mashed Potatoes

18	Broccoli Rice
19	Cashew Nut Cream
20	Mayonnaise
21	Round Roast
22	Pumpkin Soup
23	Fresh Pea Soup
24	Corn Soup
25	Avocado Sandwich
26	Vegetable Juice
27	Riso Venere Pyramid, Sautéed Shrimp, Black Squid Ink Sauce (Chef Gualtiero Marchesi)
28	Whisked Barley with Spinach and Ginger Creamy Sauce, Warm Fish Stew (Chef Fabrizio Tesse)

ONION QUICHE

Ingredients:
5 large onions sliced thin
1 tablespoon of butter
½ teaspoon of oregano
½ cup of water (4 oz)
1 package of cream cheese (8 oz)
2 teaspoons of minced parsley
2 tablespoons of chopped black olives
3 tablespoons of grated Parmesan cheese
3 egg whites (whipped to stiff peak or "snow")
480 grams (16 oz) of wheat flour*
113 grams (4 oz) of butter
Salt to taste

Servings: 4-6 people.

Making the filling:
a) In a pan, mix the butter, onions, oregano, and salt. Cook it for 5 minutes and let it cool down.
b) In a blender mix the cream cheese and the water. In a glass bowl pour the mixture of water and cream cheese, and add the parsley, olives, and Parmesan cheese.

Making the dough:
In a medium-size baking dish, place the wheat flour* and the butter. Mix everything until the dough is smooth and even (the dough should have the consistency of damp beach sand).

Preparation:
Cover the baking dish with the dough spreading it evenly on the bottom and sides. Then add the onions (a), spreading it on top of the dough (make sure the onion filling is cold or it will dissolve the dough). Add the whipped egg whites to the cream cheese mixture (b), mixing it gently and pour everything on top of the onions. Cook in oven preheated at 350° for approximately 40 minutes. When it is golden brown, it's ready.

*This pie can also be made with rice or quinoa flour.

*Remember to use only one kind of flour/starch per meal.

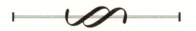

ZUCCHINI QUICHE

Ingredients:
7 small zucchinis cut in thin and wide slices
½ cup of minced black olives (4 oz)
1 cube of vegetable broth
½ onion minced
3 cloves of garlic minced
1 tablespoon of olive oil
480 grams (16 oz) of wheat flour*
113 grams (4 oz) of butter

Servings: 4-6 people.

Making the filling:
Sauté the garlic and onion in the olive oil, add the vegetable broth, the zucchinis, and the olives. Let it cook for 10 minutes. Remove from stove and let it cool.

Making the dough:
Combine wheat flour and butter. Mix it until the dough is smooth and even (the dough should have the consistency of damp beach sand), then spread it in a medium baking pan and let it bake in a preheated oven at 350° for approximately 30 minutes.

Preparation:
When the dough is baked, pour the filling into it. Sprinkle a bit of grated Parmesan cheese on top and place the dish back in the oven for 5 minutes. It's done.

*This pie can also be made with rice or quinoa flour.

*Remember to use only one kind of flour/starch per meal.

EGGPLANT QUICHE

Ingredients:
2 eggplants chopped
½ green bell pepper minced
½ red bell pepper minced
½ onion minced
3 cloves of garlic minced
2 tablespoons of minced chives
3 tablespoons of olive oil
2 tablespoons of Parmesan cheese
2 egg whites (whipped to stiff peak or "snow")
480 grams (16 oz) of wheat flour*
113 grams (4 oz) of butter

Servings: 4-6 people.

Making the filling:
Sauté the onion and the garlic in olive oil in a saucepan. When done, add the bell peppers, the eggplants, and salt. After it is cooked, add the chives. Turn the heat off, and let it cool down.

Making the dough:
Combine wheat flour and butter. Mix until the dough is smooth and even (the dough should have the consistency of damp beach sand). Then, spread it on the baking dish and bake it in a preheated oven at 350° for approximately 30 minutes.

Preparation:
When the dough is baked, pour the filling, cover it with the whipped egg whites and sprinkle the Parmesan cheese on top. Bring it back to the oven for 10 more minutes and it is ready!

*This pie can also be made with rice or quinoa flour.

* Remember to use only one kind of flour/starch per meal.

CHICKEN STROGANOFF

Ingredients:
2 lbs of boneless chicken breast cut in small squares
1 onion minced
4 cloves of garlic minced
1 tablespoon of olive oil
1 cube of chicken broth
½ cup of water (4 oz)
¼ teaspoon of oregano
3 bay leaves
4 tablespoons of tomato sauce
½ package of cream cheese (4 oz)
½ teaspoon of dried basil
1 cup of sliced mushrooms
Salt to taste

Servings: 2-4 people.

Preparation:
Marinate the chicken breast overnight with garlic, oregano, bay leaves, and salt, in a covered glass bowl. In a saucepan, heat up the olive oil and sauté the chicken pieces. Add the onion, the chicken broth, and basil. Let it cook. Separately, mix the water*, cream cheese, and tomato sauce. It should become like a cream. Add the mushrooms to the chicken**, and let it cook. Lastly, remove the bay leaves***, add the cream cheese mixture. Mix well. Do not let it boil. It's ready.

*Tip: Don't add too much water to the chicken so the cream doesn't get watered down.

**Tip: We can use the same process to make meat or shrimp stroganoff.

***Tip: Do not use oregano on fish and always remove the bay leaves before serving.

NOTE: This dish combines with any starch because it does not contain any flour.

CHICKEN SOUP

Ingredients:
1 chicken breast, clean and trimmed (preferably organic)
2 celery stalks
2 cloves of garlic, minced
¾ cup of chopped onions
2 tablespoons of extra virgin olive oil
2 bay leaves
½ cup of rice (raw and washed)
½ carrot (diced)
2 string beans (diced)
Chopped parsley to taste
Salt to taste

Servings: 4 people.

Preparation:
Season the chicken with the garlic, onion, salt, and the bay leaves the night before, until the time you start cooking. You can skip this step, but it will add more flavor to the soup. Put the olive oil and the chicken (with the seasoning) in a pressure cooker. Fry the chicken lightly, and add the celery stalks. Cover everything with water, and let it cook for 20 minutes. Remove the chicken from the pressure cooker, and reserve the broth. Shred the chicken and put it back in the pressure cooker with the broth. Add the carrots, string beans, rice, and more water, if necessary. Once everything is cooked, add the chopped parsley. Serve hot.

NOTE: This dish combines with all foods from Group A.

CREAM OF SPINACH

Ingredients:
1 bunch of spinach
½ onion minced
3 cloves of garlic minced
1 glass of water (8 oz)
½ package of cream cheese (4 oz)
1 tablespoon of olive oil
2 tablespoons of flour* (wheat, rice, or quinoa)
Salt to taste

Servings: 2-4 people.

Preparation:
Wash the spinach well and divide it in two parts.
In the blender, mix the water, cream cheese, half of the spinach, and the flour*. Chop up the rest of the spinach very small. Sauté the garlic and onion with the olive oil and add the mixture from the blender. Keep stirring until it thickens. Add the chopped spinach and cook for a couple more minutes. Serve it hot.

*Remember to use only one kind of flour/starch per meal.

CREAM OF CORN

Ingredients:
2 cans of corn (washed) or 4 ears of corn
3 cloves of garlic minced
2 tablespoons of olive oil
½ package of cream cheese (4 oz)
1 pinch of nutmeg
1 cup of water (8 oz)
2 tablespoons of flour* (wheat, rice, or quinoa)
Salt to taste

Servings: 2-4 people.

Preparation:
In the blender, mix 2 cans of corn, water, cream cheese, and flour*. Sauté the garlic in the olive oil and add the corn blend and season with salt and nutmeg. Keep stirring until it thickens. Serve it hot.

*Remember to use only one kind of flour/starch per meal.

CHAYOTE SQUASH SOUFFLÉ

Ingredients:
3 chayote squash, peeled and sliced in thick slices
½ small onion minced
3 cloves of garlic minced
1 teaspoon of oregano
2 tablespoons of olive oil
½ package of cream cheese (4 oz)
3 tablespoons of water
3 egg yolks
3 egg whites (whipped to stiff peak or "snow")
2 tablespoons of grated Parmesan cheese
Salt to taste

Servings: 2-4 people.

Preparation:
Sauté the garlic and the onion in the olive oil; Add the chayote squash, salt, and oregano and let it cook. After it is cooked, let it cool down. Mix in the blender the cream cheese, the Parmesan cheese, the egg yolks, and 3 tablespoons of water. Mix this with the chayote squash. Pour the egg whites and mix it gently. Place it all in a Pyrex baking dish greased with butter. Place it in the oven for approximately 40 minutes until golden brown. Serve hot.

NOTE: This dish combines with any starch because it does not contain any flour.

FISH SOUFFLÉ

Ingredients:
4 fish fillets (salmon, orange roughy, or tilapia)
½ of a green bell pepper minced
½ of a red bell pepper minced
1 small onion minced
3 cloves of garlic minced
2 tablespoons of olive oil
2 tablespoons of minced cilantro
1 package of cream cheese (8 oz)
3 egg yolks
3 egg whites (whipped to stiff peak or "snow")
Salt to taste

Servings: 2-4 people.

Preparation:
Cook the fish in the olive oil with garlic, onion, bell peppers, and salt. Let the fish cook in its own water; do not add water. When cooked, add the cilantro. Allow it to cook until the water dries up. Mash the fish with a fork so it will crumble. Let it cool down. Whip the cream cheese with the egg yolks and 3 tablespoons of water; add this cream to the mashed fish and mix everything. Add the whipped egg whites and mix gently. Pour everything in a Pyrex dish greased with butter and bake it in a preheated oven at 350° for approximately 40 minutes or until golden brown. It's ready to serve.

NOTE: This dish combines with any starch because it does not contain any flour.

BAKED FISH A LA COCONUT

Ingredients:
5 fish fillets, seasoned with salt only (any mild fillet such as orange roughy, halibut, sole, tilapia, etc.)
1 large onion cut in slices
2 tablespoons of capers
2 tablespoons of minced cilantro
2 tablespoons of olive oil
13 oz of coconut milk (400 ml)

Servings: 2-4 people.

Preparation:
In a Pyrex dish mix half of the onion, half of the capers, and half of the cilantro. Place the fish fillets in the Pyrex dish and cover the fish with the rest of the ingredients. Pour in the olive oil and the coconut milk. Allow it to bake at 350° for approximately 30 minutes or until the fish is golden brown. Serve it hot.

NOTE: This dish combines with any starch because it does not contain any flour.

BAKED SALMON WITH ROSEMARY (OR CAPERS)

Ingredients:
1 fillet of salmon (8 oz) seasoned with salt
3 cloves of garlic minced
3 rosemary leaves (or 1 tablespoon of capers)
2 tablespoons of olive oil

Servings: 1-2 people.

Preparation:
Mix the ingredients to make a pesto-like sauce (the quantity will vary according to the size of the salmon fillet). Be generous with the garlic and the rosemary (or capers). Spread the paste over the whole fish. Wrap the fish in aluminum foil and bake for 30 minutes at 350°. Serve it hot.

NOTE: This dish combines with any starch because it does not contain any flour.

FRESH CODFISH AND POTATO CASSEROLE

Ingredients:
4 slices of fresh codfish (not dry and salty)
1 cup of extra virgin olive oil
1 small onion cut in slices
1 tablespoon of parsley, finely chopped
3 cloves of garlic, minced
14 oz potatoes lightly cooked in salty water and sliced
Pink salt to taste
3 eggs, boiled and sliced
Green olives to taste, sliced

Servings: 4 people.

Preparation:
Heat the olive oil in a big pan and add the onions, garlic, and parsley. Sauté until the onion starts to change color. Place the sliced potatoes in the pot and leave for about 10 minutes, until they start to fry. Cover the bottom of a large baking dish with the potatoes, and place the fish slices on top. Season with salt. The layers should not be too thick. Pour the contents of the frying pan on top of the casserole and place it in the oven for 15 to 20 minutes, or until the fish is cooked. Remove it from the oven and garnish with the sliced eggs and olives.

NOTE: Since potatoes (Group B), are used in this dish, other starches should not be added. However, potato chips, French fries, and other forms of preparation of potatoes would combine, as well as any other foods from Group A can be included in this meal.

SHRIMP HUNGARIAN STYLE
(A specialty from Rufino's Restaurant, São Paulo, Brazil)

Ingredients:
2 lbs pink shrimp, peeled and washed
8 oz cream cheese
1 tablespoon of paprika
Pink salt to taste
1 lb potatoes, cooked and sliced
1 tablespoon of butter
¼ cup of water
3 garlic cloves, minced
1 tablespoon of extra virgin olive oil

Servings: 4 people.

Preparation:
Cook the sliced potatoes in a pot, covered with salty water. Place the olive oil and the butter in a pan, and add the shrimp and the garlic. Fry until the shrimp change color. Place the cooked potatoes in a baking dish, and cover with the fried shrimp. In a blender, combine the cream cheese, water, and one tablespoon of butter. Pour this mixture over the shrimp, sprinkle with paprika, and cover with aluminum foil. Place it in a preheated oven at 425° F until it starts to bubble. Remove the aluminum foil and bake until golden. *Bon appétit!*

NOTE: As potatoes are used in this dish (Group B), other starches should not be added. However, potatoes prepared in other ways, and any foods from Group A, can be added to this meal.

SHRIMP AND POTATO COMBO

Ingredients:
1 lb of potatoes
2 eggs
½ package of cream cheese (4 oz)
¼ cup of water (2 oz)
1 tablespoon of minced cilantro
3 tablespoons of grated Parmesan cheese
1 lb of clean shrimp
2 tablespoons of olive oil
1 onion minced
2 cloves of garlic minced
2 tomatoes peeled and minced
½ green bell pepper minced
200 ml of coconut milk (7 oz)
2 tablespoons of potato starch diluted in 200 ml of water (7 oz)
Salt to taste

Servings: 2-4 people.

Preparing the potatoes:
Cook the potatoes. When done mash the potatoes and mix in the eggs and the cilantro. In a blender mix the water and cream cheese. Add the cream cheese blend to the mashed potatoes and mix well. Let it sit.

Preparing the filling:
Sauté the garlic and the onion in olive oil; add the bell pepper and the tomato and let it cook for 5 minutes. Add the shrimp seasoned with only salt. Let it cook until the shrimp

turn pink-colored. Add the coconut milk and the diluted potato starch to the shrimp in the pan and stir it until it thickens.

Assembling it:
In a Pyrex dish greased with butter, spread half of the mashed potato mix evenly. Pour the shrimp and then cover it with the rest of the potato mix. Sprinkle the Parmesan cheese and bake it in a preheated oven at 350° for 30 minutes and it will be ready to serve.

NOTE: Since potato is the starch of choice for this meal, French fries or potato chips would be OK. However, include no other starch such as breads, beans, rice, corn flour, etc. (Group B).

SHRIMP LINGUINE

Ingredients:
8 oz linguine
Olive oil
3 cloves of garlic, minced
16 medium shrimp, peeled and washed
Pink salt to taste
A handful of fresh basil, chopped

Servings: 4 people.

Preparing the pasta:
Cook the pasta in plenty of salted water until al dente. Drain and put aside. In a big pan, place the olive oil and the garlic. Sauté until the garlic is lightly golden. Add the shrimp and fry until they change color and cook inside. Season with salt. Combine the pasta with a little of its cooking water, and the fried shrimp with garlic. Sprinkle with chopped basil and serve.

NOTE: This dish combines with other foods made from wheat (Group B), and all foods in Group A.

GLUTEN-FREE QUICHE

Ingredients:
1 bunch of kale, finely chopped
1 big ball of mozzarella, sliced
3 cloves of garlic, minced
1 tablespoon of cream cheese or cashew nut cream
2 eggs
1 tablespoon of coconut oil
Pink salt to taste
3 oz water

Servings: 4 people.

Preparation:
Sauté the garlic in the coconut oil. Add the chopped kale and let it wither. Add the cream cheese (or cashew nut cream) and the water. Put aside. Grease a baking dish with coconut oil and place the kale mixture in it. Whisk the two eggs and pour over the mixture. Garnish with the mozzarella slices and cover with aluminum foil, without closing on the sides. Place the dish in a preheated oven at 350°F for 20 minutes, or until the eggs are cooked.

NOTE: This dish combines with any starch in Group B, as well as all meats and vegetables in Group A.

MASHED POTATOES

Ingredients:
5 medium potatoes
1 tablespoon of butter
¼ package of cream cheese (2 oz)
¼ glass of water (2 oz)
Salt to taste

Servings: 2-4 people.

Preparation:
Peel and cook the potatoes. Blend the cream cheese and the water. After cooked, mash the potatoes well and add the butter, the blended cream cheese, and salt. It's ready. Enjoy!

NOTE: You may eat mashed potatoes (Group B) with meat, poultry, or fish, and/or vegetables (Group A).

BROCCOLI RICE

Ingredients:
1 cup of white rice, washed and drained
2 cloves of garlic, minced
1 tablespoon of coconut oil
4 cups of finely chopped broccoli, including the stalks
2½ cups of water
Salt to taste

Servings: 4 people.

Preparation:
Sauté the minced garlic in the coconut oil, add the rice, and let it braise for a while. Add the broccoli and the water, season with salt, and let it cook on medium heat. When it starts to boil, cover the pot, reduce the heat, and cook until the water has completely dried out.

NOTE: You can serve the Broccoli Rice (Group B) with any of the foods in Group A.

CASHEW NUT CREAM

Ingredients:
6 oz cashew nuts, raw and unsalted
1½ cups of water

Servings: 2-4 portions.

Preparation:
Cover the cashew nuts with water and let them soak overnight. On the following day, drain the nuts and place them in a blender, adding another cup of fresh water. Blend until smooth.

NOTE: This cream of cashews is a great substitute for cream cheese in stovetop recipes.

MAYONNAISE

Ingredients:
3 egg yolks cooked
3 egg yolks raw
Extra virgin olive oil
Salt to taste

Servings: 2-4 portions.

Preparation:
In a blender, place the egg yolks (the cooked and the raw) and one tablespoon of olive oil. Blend until smooth. If necessary, add more olive oil while blending, and salt to taste. Let it cool in the refrigerator before serving.

NOTE: Serve this mayonnaise with salads.

ROUND ROAST

Ingredients:
1 (4 ½ pound) round roast
1 onion chopped
3 garlic cloves minced
1 medium carrot
½ teaspoon of oregano
3 bay leaves
4 tablespoons of olive oil
2 glasses of water (8 oz each)
Salt to taste

Servings: 4-6 people.

Preparation:
Wash the meat and place it in a glass bowl with onions, garlic, oregano, bay leaves, and salt. Poke a hole through the meat with a knife and stick the carrot in it. Cover the bowl and let it marinate for at least 8 hours in the refrigerator.

Heat up the olive oil in a pan and place the meat in it. (Wipe off the ingredients with your hand before placing the meat in the hot oil; the carrot stays in.) Move the roast around the pan until it acquires an even color all over it. Then, place the ingredients back into the pan with the meat (except for the bay leaves) and let them cook a little to a brown color; it will add flavor. Then add the water and let it cook for about 45 minutes, turning the roast once in a while. Make sure the water does not dry out completely. If you need to add a bit more, it's OK. By scraping the bottom of the pan once in a while with a wooden spoon, you will end up with the cooked ingredients and the meat juice as a flavorful sauce for the roast.

NOTE: This dish would combine with any one starch: rice, pasta, potato, etc., (Group B) and any vegetable (Group A).

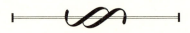

PUMPKIN SOUP

Ingredients:
2 lbs pumpkin
½ tablespoon of butter or olive oil
½ onion, finely chopped
1 clove of garlic, minced
34 oz hot water
1 tablespoon of cream cheese
Salt to taste

Servings: 2-4 people.

Preparation:
Wash the pumpkin under running tap water. On a cutting board, peel it and cut it in half. Remove the seeds and dice the pumpkin. Melt the butter in a medium size pot and sauté the onion in the butter until it changes color. Add the minced garlic and stir for over one minute. Place the diced pumpkin in the pan, and sauté for another minute. Add the hot water and cover the pot. Let it cook for about 20 minutes after it starts to boil, or until the pumpkin is tender. Remove from the heat and put the pumpkin cubes in a blender. Blend while adding the cooking water, little by little, until you reach the desired consistency. Put the pumpkin cream back in the pot, over low heat. Add the cream cheese and stir until it melts. It is ready!

NOTE: This dish combines with any starch (Group B), as well as the foods in Group A. It goes very well with the Avocado Sandwich.

FRESH PEA SOUP

Ingredients:
1 bag of fresh peas
½ white onion, chopped
1 clove of garlic, minced
1 tablespoon of parsley, finely chopped
16 oz water
1 tablespoon of coconut oil
A small tip of ginger (optional)

Servings: 4 people.

Preparation:
In a pot over medium heat, sauté the onion and the garlic with the coconut oil, until it withers a little. Wash the peas, place them in the pot, and stir for a while. Add the water and let it boil. Remove from the stove and put everything in a blender. Blend until smooth. If desired, add the ginger. Finally, add the parsley and blend it again. Serve hot.

NOTE: This dish combines with any starch (Group B), and the foods in Group A. The Avocado Sandwich is a great complement for this soup.

CORN SOUP

Ingredients:
1 dozen ears of sweet corn
Olive oil
Salt to taste

Observation: You'll need a juicer for this one.

Servings: 1-2 people.

Preparation:
Shuck the corn and shave the kernels into a bowl. Put the kernels through the juicer. Put the "corn juice" into a pan and cook it on a low flame stirring nonstop with a wooden spoon so the corn juice does not get stuck to the bottom of the pan. When it starts to boil, it's done. Add olive oil and salt to taste.

NOTE: You can complete this meal with a grilled Monterey Jack cheese sandwich on sourdough or whole grain bread.

AVOCADO SANDWICH

Ingredients:
1 ripe avocado
2 slices of whole grain wheat bread
1 tablespoon of raw cashews
1 tablespoon of olive oil
1 coffee spoon of wheat germ
1 thin slice of onion (optional)
2 leaves of lettuce washed and dried
Salt to taste

Servings: 1 person.

Preparation:
Toast the bread. Wash, cut open, and mash the avocado with a fork. Add olive oil and salt to taste. The onion slice can be raw or sautéed in a few drops of olive oil. Spread the avocado on the toast, sprinkle the wheat germ, add the onion, top it with the leaves of lettuce, and cap the sandwich with the other slice of toast. Try it with all the ingredients, and then adapt it to your own preferences. If one isn't enough, make two.

NOTE: This sandwich would combine well with the vegetable juice.

VEGETABLE JUICE

Ingredients:
1 medium cucumber
3 leaves of kale
2 radishes
3 sticks of celery
1 stick of broccoli
1 bell pepper
1 green onion
1 small tip of ginger (optional)
6 carrots

Servings: 1-2 people.

Preparation:
Wash all vegetables thoroughly, using any of the vegetable wash products readily available. Peel the cucumber, the ginger, and the carrots, and then pass all the vegetables through a juicer. Feel free to add additional vegetables to the mix or modify the proportions to your liking. If you can, always use organic vegetables.

NOTE: This vegetable juice combines well with the avocado sandwich.

Italian Chef Gualtiero Marchesi is considered to be the founder of modern Italian cuisine. We are honored that he would share this special recipe with us. Grazie Maestro!

RISO VENERE PYRAMID, SAUTÉED SHRIMP, BLACK SQUID INK SAUCE

Ingredients:
¾ lbs of riso venere (black rice)
black squid ink sauce (*)
16 red shrimp
2 oz of small calamari
½ oz of fresh ginger
1 oz of basil
White celery leaves
Extra virgin olive oil
Salt

Black Squid Ink Sauce (*)

Ingredients:
.95 oz of butter
.95 oz of black squid ink
.45 oz of onions, chopped
1.8 oz of water

Servings: 4 people.

Preparation of Ink Sauce:
Sauté the onions in the butter. Add the water and the black squid ink. Bring to a boil. Pass through a sieve and make a reduction to the desired consistency. Put aside.

Directions:
Cook rice in hot salted water. In the meantime, in a pan, sauté the shrimp (previously cut vertically) and the small calamari with a little olive oil, without salt.
Now prepare the sauce with the black squid ink as explained above, and leave aside. For the basil sauce, emulsify the basil with the rest of the oil and leave aside. Grease the pyramid molds with a little bit of oil. Fill them with the boiled rice seasoned with ginger and some white celery leaves. When it is time to serve, flip the pyramid in the middle of the plate and surround it with both the sauces and alternate one shrimp and one calamari around the plate.

Chef Fabrizio Tesse, a Michelin Star recipient, has prepared this recipe 100% Gracie Way compliant. Bravissimo!

WHISKED BARLEY WITH SPINACH AND GINGER CREAMY SAUCE, WARM FISH STEW

Ingredients:
9 oz of barley
10.5 oz of fresh spinach
1 oz of fresh ginger
10.5 oz of mixed fresh fish (redfish, mullet, bonito)
.35 oz of butter
.7 oz of Parmigiano Reggiano
17 oz of fresh vegetable broth
Aromatic herbs, basil sprouts, red beet sprouts, burnet herb
1 tablespoon of extra virgin olive oil

Servings: 4 people.

Preparation:
Wash the barley under water, dry it, and toast in a casserole dish. Once at temperature, add the hot broth, and then finish cooking it. Previously cook the spinach in boiling water and after two minutes cool it down in water and ice. Squeeze and blend with the fresh ginger and one tablespoon of extra virgin olive oil. Once the barley is cooked, whisk it with the spinach and ginger sauce, adding butter and Parmigiano. Cut the fish in small pieces, steam it for a few minutes, and add salt.

The Plate:
Place the barley on a large plate and add the stewed fish. Garnish the fish with the aromatic herbs.